HEAL

HEAL

Your Path to Thriving

DEB HARRELL, ND

XULON PRESS

Xulon Press
2301 Lucien Way #415
Maitland, FL 32751
407.339.4217
www.xulonpress.com

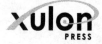

Paperback ISBN-13: 978-1-6628-3409-7
Ebook ISBN-13: 978-1-6628-3412-7

I dedicate this book to my beautiful friend Gigi Honeycutt, who got her heavenly promotion on September 27, 2021. Your courage, faith, and persistence will forever be a reminder to me to never give up. I carry on with my mission in honor of you. I look forward to seeing you again my friend. You will be missed!

TABLE OF CONTENTS

FOREWORD

I REMEMBER THE first time I met Deb. I was a Critical Care Registered Nurse at the time and new to the arena of prevention and "food as medicine." I was so hungry to learn. Dr. Deb came to the rescue! She was eager to help and generous with her time and resources as she taught me the basics of whole food nutrition and the power of the body to heal. She even invited me to her home for healthy cooking demonstrations. As a result, my lifestyle started transforming from a sedentary fast-food junkie to an active, thriving, intentional plant-based foodie! That was over twenty-five years ago! Deb was also a valuable buddy to me in my weight-loss journey, supporting me all the way. I couldn't have done it without her love and encouragement! We became very good friends and to this day, even though I have since become a Naturopathic Doctor and Counselor of Natural Health, she is my number one go-to for all things health and wellness. Why? She has been on this health journey for decades and has invested time and money into becoming an expert in her field. But most importantly, she lives what she teaches with passion and purpose! In her well thought-out-book, Dr. Deb will walk the reader from the mindset needed for a positive lifestyle change, to why and how to cleanse and detoxify your body and your home, and to how to get started making proactive food choices while creating a lifestyle that will sustain vitality well into your nineties (or beyond)! This book is written like an easy-to-follow-and-apply tutorial for anyone seeking health, vitality, resources, and answers. I am honored to recommend *HEAL* to my family, friends, and clients as I am confident this will be their go-to resource for proactive health and wellness.

Carol Watson, RN, ND, Life & Body Confidence Coach, Speaker, and Trainer **www.tcDrCarol.com**

INTRODUCTION

MY STORY

"Truth has no special time of its own. Its hour is now – always."

Albert Schweitzer

HELLO, MY NAME is Deb. I am passionate about eliminating suffering in this world. I have lofty goals and big ideals. I'm an eternal optimist. I'm on a mission to make a difference in our troubled, unhealthy world. I do not believe in coincidences and therefore I believe this book is for you since it's in your hands. You did not just stumble upon it. You are here for a reason. My prayer is that the Creator of the universe speaks to you through these words and as a result, you will never be the same.

I'm recognized by many as an expert and someone who can help you overcome disease processes. I'm honored by that, but what many people don't know is that I have struggled with self-sabotage in my life. I have overcome some tough challenges, including a duodenal ulcer, came out on the other side successfully, and I want to give you the benefit of the things I have learned. Plus, I have had a lot of education and experience concerning how to get and stay healthy using a holistic approach. I help sick and tired people change their lifestyles so they can live a life of thriving and not just surviving. I'm like a genie in a bottle for people serious about getting and staying well. I like to think of myself as the Dave Ramsey[1] of health.

I have worked with many people with health challenges, including late-stage cancer. I have witnessed the power of the principles I share with you here. God created your body as a self-healing mechanism. Every cell of your body is programmed to heal itself if given the right environment. Symptoms are nothing more than your body's attempt to get well.

My path along this journey has been anything but straight, but I have learned that when things happen and feel random, in hindsight they usually have a purpose. Even journeys to the darkest places will serve us if we grow through those times. I believe we will look back at our lives and see this beautiful tapestry with every piece fitting together beautifully.

When I was eighteen years old and in my first year of college, I became a vegetarian because I did not like eating animals. I love animals and can't stand the horror they go through to get to our plate. I began my plant-based journey however as a junk food vegetarian. No animals were suffering from my food choices, but I was. Many ethical vegetarians or vegans avoid animal products but fill up on processed junk food. Unfortunately, they don't radiate the health that a plant-based diet can afford because they are, like most Americans, choosing edible food-like substances instead of whole food (more on this later).

I was blessed with motherhood at twenty-five years old, which caused me to reevaluate my predominantly junk-food diet. I wanted to feed that beautiful little miracle everything possible to ensure her health. I switched to whole-wheat flour, natural sweeteners, and more whole plant foods. However, we

---

[1]   Dave Ramsey has shared practical answers to life's tough money questions since 1992. www.DaveRamsey.com

continued eating dairy and eggs. When my daughter Cristina was in first grade, she was sick a lot. We spent a lot of time in the pediatrician's office. At the end of her first-grade year, the doctor recommended that we remove her tonsils and adenoids. I immediately screeched on the brakes because I couldn't bear the thought of my baby going into surgery. Although I was not a believer then, I had this feeling that everything that God put in the body must have some purpose and it made little sense to cut out body parts. I asked my chiropractor for his advice, and he recommended getting her off dairy, doing lymphatic drainage massages that he taught us, and taking her to a homeopathic doctor. Homeopathy is the treatment of disease by minute doses of natural substances that in a healthy person would produce symptoms of the disease.[2] It's been around for over two-hundred years in Europe and is very effective in helping the body fight illness. It gives a nudge to the immune system, so to speak. I've found it to work beautifully for many different maladies.

We did all those things, and Cristina still has her tonsils and adenoids thirty-eight years later. I am so grateful because they are key components to the immune system. Tonsils and adenoids are often referred to as our last line of defense against cancer. That experience with my daughter was my launch into the alternative medicine world. I learned that the right food is our best medicine, and the wrong food is an enemy to our health. God used that experience with my daughter to get me on the path to my purpose.

I then read the book by bestselling author, John Robbins, titled *Diet for a New America*[3]. That book rocked my world and caused my husband and I to give up animal products altogether. John

---

[2]   https://www.homeopathycenter.org/
what-is-homeopathy/#whatishomeopathy

[3]   John Robbins, *Diet for a New America, How Your Food Choices Affect Your Health, Happiness, and the Future of Life on Earth*, (Tiburon, CA: HJ Kramer, Inc., 1987), www.johnrobbins.info

was the heir to the Baskin Robbins fortune and walked away from the family business because of what ice cream does to people's health. He spent several years researching for the book which looks at animal food consumption and its impact on our health, the animals, and the environment. I highly recommend that book, which is now a twenty-five-year anniversary edition. It changed my life, and it can yours too.

After reading *Diet for a New America*, I began "preaching" to everyone I saw on the dangers of animal products. I had a passion well up inside of me to get the message out to anyone and everyone who would listen. I was overzealous in my approach, but my intent was to help people avoid suffering caused by their food choices. I began educating myself more on the value of using food as medicine.

Soon after reading that book, I recommitted my life to God and got involved in a local non-denominational church. I saw an attitude in church that you pray over your food and believe that God will bless it. Despite that being nowhere in scripture (asking God to bless a meal), it just did not make sense to me. Giving thanks for the food, yes, but asking God to bless it, especially when it was edible food-like substances He never meant for us to eat seems completely inappropriate, doesn't it? "Dear Lord, please remove the cholesterol, nitrates, pesticides, sugar, hormones, and saturated fat from this 'food' and make it nourishing to my body." I mean, that is not what we say, but it is the reality of the prayer. I just don't believe God is going to "bless it for our nourishment." This attitude bothered me as I witnessed the prayer list for sick people grow longer and longer at our church.

During this time a young lady in her twenties in our church who loved God and trusted Him with all her heart got diagnosed with cancer. Unfortunately, she lost that battle and went to Heaven far too soon, in my opinion. She chose the traditional medical route of treatment. During one of her stays in the hospital, our pastor ran into a doctor who gave him the book titled *Why Christians Get Sick*[4] by George Malkmus, founder of Hallelujah Acres and Back to the Garden Health Ministry (www. hacres.com.) George was healed of cancer using God's original food—plant foods. Genesis 1:29, NIV translation says, "Then God said, 'I give you every seed-bearing plant on the face of the whole earth and every tree that has fruit with seed in it. They will be yours for food.'"

I was so excited to get hold of this book. Finally, I found someone who could relate to my frustrations of seeing people perish. I called George Malkmus after reading his book. We had a long conversation and discovered that we had both gone plant-based the same year. I had a new passion—reaching the church with this message.

In 1996, I attended Hallelujah Acres and became certified as a Back to the Garden Health Minister. I was ecstatic! I met some amazing people who were on the same path I was. We all had a passion to make a difference in people's lives.

After the young lady I mentioned passed away, our church hosted George Malkmus to come and give his life-saving message. It was a splendid night, and many people embraced the changes he recommended. Unfortunately, most of those people did not stick with the changes. Because I was a trained health minister and had been living the lifestyle for twenty years at that point, I began teaching classes at the church on how to implement a plant-based lifestyle. That was my first teaching experience, and it was a scary one as I was not a public speaker. My passion to help others propelled me to do the classes despite my fear.

That night at the talk someone asked me to call a woman they knew who had just been diagnosed with cancer. Her name was

---

[4]   George Malkmus, *Why Christians Get Sick*, (Destiny Image Publishers, 2005)

Gigi and I remember pulling up in front of her house thinking, "What if I share this plan with her and she dies?" I immediately felt as if God spoke to me saying, "You are just the messenger. What she does with the info is between me and her." That gave me the peace I needed to proceed. I walked into Gigi's house that night and found a bunch of kids running around and a woman who looked frazzled and scared. She had just been released from the hospital from having a breast lumpectomy. She had not received good news–stage three going into stage four breast cancer.

I had many conversations with Gigi over the next month, encouraging her to seek God's will for the situation and providing her guidance on using food as medicine for her condition. We talked about what it would involve should she go the natural route–juicing, lots of raw organic fruits and veggies, detoxing her home, dealing with her emotions, etc. She took a month to decide, and she chose the holistic route, despite her doctors telling her she would die if she did not do their treatments. Gigi survived that battle twenty-five years ago. However, I am saddened to say that she just lost a second battle with breast cancer yesterday, after fighting valiantly for the past two and a half years. Gigi regretfully admitted to me that she abandoned the healthy ways that healed her in her first cancer battle. She also waited until the cancer had progressed significantly this second time before doing anything about it. Gigi wrote a testimony for this book about a year ago, and it is below. Based on many conversations I had with her these past few years, I am certain she would want me to add this to her testimony: "Don't put off until tomorrow taking care of yourself. It might just be too late. Make self-care a priority today and stick with it, even if you feel well and think you no longer must be proactive. You always must be proactive. You are worth it." I will be forever grateful for Gigi's life and friendship. Her healing came on the other side of eternity, and I will see her again!

STORY TIME: GIGI HONEYCUTT

"I have known Deb Harrell for twenty-five years and she truly cares for people. Her dedication and love for me during my two battles with breast cancer were life changing for me. I have personally witnessed that Deb lives and breathes everything written in this book. There is truth and wisdom written here and I recommend you read every word. This book will encourage you and help guide you in the right direction to become both physically and emotionally healthy. Implement these modalities Deb writes about here and just wait to see what God can do in your life! Be blessed!"

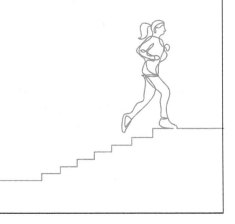

Through attending the Hallelujah Acres health minister reunions every year, I met some great doctor health crusaders: Dr. Loraine Day who healed her cancer using the power of plants (www.drday.com), Dr. Francisco Contreras from the Oasis of Hope Hospital in Mexico where they treat cancer alternatively (www.oasisofhope.com), and Dr. Joel Robbins, (http://drjoelrobbins.com) who has a holistic clinic in Oklahoma. I also got to hear Charlotte Gerson speak. Charlotte was Max Gerson's daughter who carried on his legacy heading up the Gerson Clinic in Mexico (www.gerson.org.) I learned so much from these amazing wellness warriors and owe each a debt of gratitude!

Over the years, I have continued my education learning as much as possible on how to equip people to prevent and heal disease. You will hear about a few of the other people I have helped later. I am always honored to be a small part of a person's journey! Think of this book as a sort of virtual consultation with me, where you can learn the path I recommend for you to thrive—body, soul, and spirit.

Please know that it is easier to prevent than reverse disease. I encourage you to start now on a healthy lifestyle because your future health starts right now! You don't always feel disease developing inside the body, so you cannot go on what you feel. Be proactive to prevent any future issues and/or to correct some things that might be moving in the wrong direction.

We live in a fast-paced world that has become increasingly more toxic. We are largely overfed but undernourished. We fill up on "edible food-like substances"[5] instead of authentic food. It is more important now than ever to practice self-care. I will not go into all the scientific research showing how a whole-food plant-based lifestyle is your best bet to live in vitality and

---

[5]   Michael Pollan, *In Defense of Food, An Eater's Manifesto,* (Penguin Books, 2009)

health, because many health professionals have done a superb job with that. I provide my suggested reading list if you need more convincing, or are the type that likes to read the science. I feel my job here is to merely guide you on how-to live-in health from a practical standpoint. This workbook will serve as a virtual classroom with me. And because wellness is a matter of body, soul, and spirit, this is a holistic guide incorporating nutrition and the other components to health as shown on the HEAL compass on the cover.

My instructor in the naturopath program taught there were only two reasons for dis-ease—ignorance and laziness. I am equipping you in this workbook with the knowledge you need to live a healthy, whole-food plant-based lifestyle. You can no longer claim ignorance. It's up to you to do your part and take care of the laziness reason. Dr. Robbins also taught that there are only two causes of disease—nutritional deficiencies and toxicity. Your main health goal should be to get the nutrients in and the toxins out. Make that your mantra—nutrients in, toxins out. You can distill any recommendation through those two filters. Will this get nutrients in my body and toxins out? I show you how to do both in this book.

I provide you a chapter with recipes that I know you will love—recipes that will nourish your body and help you live in peak health. I love to cook for people. Just ask anyone who knows me. I suppose my interest in cooking began when a friend gave me a Betty Crocker kids cookbook for my eighth birthday party. I loved trying the simple recipes contained within when I was able to persuade my mother to allow me to invade the kitchen. I admit that I'm a decent cook these days. I simply go into the kitchen and take what I have on hand and create something delicious. Trust me when I tell you I've come a long way in this department. My husband jokes that during our early married years he always knew when dinner was ready by when the smoke detector went off. Although that happened some, I'm quite certain he exaggerates! I've collected recipes over the forty-plus years I've been plant-based that most everyone likes, even major meat eaters. I encourage you to try them all and find out your favorites. I also encourage you to get a three-ring binder and collect your favorite plant-based recipes from the resources I have listed for you in Chapter 6. Or you can simply save them on your phone.

I assure you that your destiny is to live in health and vitality. However, your participation is required to make this a reality. I call it the divine-human partnership for your health. I encourage you to view the journey as a fun adventure. It's not about what you need to give up, but about what you get to experience—new flavors, new habits, extra energy, and health. Let the journey begin!

TIME TO SMILE

June showed up at work on Monday morning with both of her ears bandaged. Her boss Ellie asked, "Oh my gosh, what happened to you?" June answered, "Well I was ironing the other day and the phone rang and I answered the iron instead of the phone." In disbelief Ellie replied, "Well what in the world happened to the other ear?" June glumly answered, "They called back!"

I often begin my seminars with this joke to highlight what insanity looks like. We often define insanity as doing the same thing over-and-over again and expecting a different result. Unfortunately, that is often what we do with our health. We keep repeating the same bad habits and somehow expect a different result. Hopefully this book will help you break the insanity loop and reclaim your health!

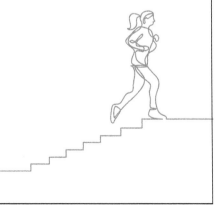

CHAPTER 1

ENEMIES OF YOUR HEALTH

"The smarter we become the sicker we become, because we are looking for cures instead of causes."

Joel Robbins, ND, DC

WHY DO MOST people who receive bad news of a degenerative disease diagnosis not stick with a healthy lifestyle, when they know beyond any doubt that it is in their best interest to do so? Why do most people start healthy new year's resolutions only to abandon them shortly after starting? Why do people carry on with their addictions despite it ruining their lives and those they love? What are these apparent enemies to your health?

ENEMY #1–YOU

Oftentimes you are your biggest enemy, aren't you? Especially when it comes to your health. Many times, people won't stick with healthy habits because of emotional hurts that still need healing. People soothe those hurts by self-medicating with food, alcohol, drugs, sex, overworking, control, etc. I have done that in my younger years with several of these things. I can relate! Been there, done that, got the T-shirt–multiple t-shirts. I thank God I'm still alive today because I should not be. I can remember waking up one morning while in my twenties, after a night of drinking and partying, and asking, "Did I wreck my car last night? I kind of remember that I did." I went down to the street and sure enough, the entire side of my Datsun Honeybee (I know this shows my age) had a very large gash in it. Dang, really Deb?

My older eighteen-year-old brother Bobby died in a car accident where all the boys were drinking, including the driver. Bobby was the only one who was seriously injured. I was eleven, and it rocked my family's world. You will hear more about that later. One would think that kind of life-altering experience would have caused me to never drive and drink. Unfortunately, it did not! Why? Because I had emotional pains I was trying to soothe with alcohol and therefore reason flew out the window. Emotional wounds that are unhealed will cause us to self-sabotage, and that's what I was doing. I often wonder why my life was spared and not my brother's. I realize and accept that there are many questions I won't have an answer to this side of eternity. Although I don't know the answer, I trust the One who does.

Unfortunately, in today's world we want relief without responsibility. We want to go about our merry way and expect someone to rescue us; we want the medical profession, or God, to heal us miraculously. I believe we are to be in a partnership with God concerning our lives, and our health. The church teaches Biblical stewardship of finances, relationships, etc., but most churches neglect to teach stewardship of the body that carries us around on planet earth. That is a sad thing, and I believe one reason the prayer list for sick people is so long.

You must accept personal responsibility for your health. It is your responsibility and yours alone. It is not your spouse's, your kid's, your pastor's, your doctor's, or even God's responsibility.

It is yours. Period. The faster you accept that fact, the better off you will be. This is good news because who is the one and only person on the planet you can control? Yep, the one in the mirror staring back at you. So yay, good news is you have the power. Take it back! Taking personal responsibility eliminates the temptation to make excuses.

Another thing we do is gamble. Yep, I said that right. But you are saying to me right now that you don't go to casinos, or play online poker, or play the ponies. OK, that's great! You will save yourself a lot of money and heartache by not gambling with money. But you gamble every day with your health and your life when you don't take personal responsibility for your habits. Each time you continue eating that junk food, smoking that cigarette, forgoing exercise, drinking too many alcoholic beverages, not drinking enough water, etc., you are gambling. You can either be a gambler or an investor. It is your choice. Are you willing to gamble—take that chance—that your bad habits or lack of good habits will not eventually catch up with you? Or will you take back personal responsibility for your health and invest in you? You have started the investing pro- cess by investing in and reading this book. Reach around and give yourself a pat on the back. You have taken step one as an investor. Congratulations! Now the next step is applying the recommendations in this book. Your future health starts right now! Will you invest in it to make sure you get a good return? From now on, I encourage you to adopt an investor mentality and drop the gambling because gambling never pays off in the long run, while investing does. You are worth it! Your family is worth it!

ENEMY #2-THE FLOCK MENTALITY

The second potential enemy of your health is the flock men- tality. I love birds and I spend a lot of time observing them. God has used birds many times to teach me "aha" life lessons. Birds of a feather flock together, as the saying coined by William

Turner goes. They do what the other members of the flock do. I feed ducks and Canadian geese in the back of my house daily. If one member of the gaggle (flock of geese) suddenly takes off and starts flying, the others do the same. There is no apparent reason to me why they suddenly do that.

We people have our own flocks, which are good for us–most of the time. We are created to live in community with others. We however have a highly functioning brain and don't rely on instincts, as animals do. We, out of all the creatures on this earth, are the only species endowed with the power to choose. That can be good news, or it can be bad news.

I see people abandon their healthy lifestyle because they want to "fit in" with their "flock." This is especially prevalent in the church. People don't want to stand out in their small groups or congregation by eating differently. "I mean, if my pastor eats certain things, why shouldn't I?", they reason. Never mind that your pastor is not the picture of vitality and health. The simple fact is that people don't want to differ from their flock. It is said that you will have similar habits to the five closest people to you. You typically eat, think, and act like those you hang out with. It is human nature.

God created you to be your own unique, one-of-a-kind self. Be true to your convictions and lead the flock! I have not eaten meat since January of 1976. I have successfully dined with many people, although they were eating meat. You can stand up and be different and still enjoy being a part of a flock. Just don't allow the flock to influence you in the wrong way. You influence them with your healthy example. My life quote is by Albert Schweitzer, "Example is not the main thing in influencing others, it's the only thing."[6] Many people have come back to me over time and asked for my advice after watching

---

[6]   https://www.quotes.net/quote/38643

my example for years. Wouldn't you love to influence your flock to be healthier?

Many cite not wanting to offend others as their reason to not be different with eating habits. You can avoid offending people by being true to yourself, by accepting them as they are in their journey, and by keeping your mouth closed unless asked. I have had to learn this over the years because I want to shout this message from the rooftops. I have such a passion to see people get and stay well. I learned however that I can only help those who want help. I have learned that lesson through much anguish and buckets of tears because often those closest to me have rejected my advice. Even Jesus had that problem! He said, "A prophet is not without honor except in his hometown and in his own household."[7] I remind myself of that a lot when I feel I have life-saving info for people I love and care about and they don't want it.

You can also easily go to other people's houses to eat without offending them. If you had a gluten allergy such as celiac disease, would you not let your hosts know beforehand, or would you eat gluten and suffer the consequences later? Of course, you would let them know and it would not offend the host. You can do the same thing concerning meat and animal products. You tell your host you are on a special diet for health reasons (and you are!). I let people know that a salad and baked potato are all I need for dinner. I need nothing fancy. The whole point of getting together is the fellowship anyway!

The lack of focus on teaching the importance of physical stewardship or looking one hundred percent to the Bible for guidance and ignoring valid science, has led to a situation that is less than appealing for the church. Several studies show that Christians don't fare as well as non-Christians (except for

---

[7]   Matthew 13:57, NIV

Seventh Day Adventists that incorporate a lot of what I suggest in this book) concerning their health.

Let's look at some results of these studies. A 2011 Northwestern University study tracked 2,433 men and women for eighteen years. They found that young adults that attended church or a Bible study at least once a week were fifty percent more likely to be obese than their non-church-going counterparts.[8] Gulp! A 2006 Purdue University study found that there was a correlation between religious participation and being overweight, with those of the Baptist denomination having a larger percentage of overweight people. The study found that Seventh Day Adventist and Mormons evaded this dilemma, which makes sense as both religions teach on physical stewardship of the body.[9]

Trust me, there is plenty of obesity and lack of health with non-churchgoers as well. The reality is that we live in a culture of excess, and we tend to adapt our behaviors to our tribe (those people we do life with.) This has been seen time and again when foreigners come to America and adopt our bad food choices. They start suffering the same ill effects as their American neighbors. My sister Karen taught ESL (English as a Second Language) in high school and often saw this with her students.

Let me be clear, being overweight or obese is a health issue, not a cosmetic one. I never want to shame anyone for being overweight. Emotional issues are one of the many reasons to have excess weight, as I mentioned earlier. Food addiction is an actual thing. It does not differ from alcoholism or any other addiction, except that in food addiction, it is impossible

---

[8]   https://www.ncbi.nlm.nih.gov/pmc/articles/PMC3310238/ Coronary Artery Risk Development in Young Adults (CARDIA) multi-center study, supported by the National Heart, Lung and Blood Institute

[9]   https://www.ncbi.nlm.nih.gov/pmc/articles/PMC3358928/

to avoid the substance you are addicted to like you can with drugs and alcohol. Many times, addiction results from trying to soothe an unresolved hurt in your life. I come from a family of alcoholics, so I have had experience with addicts my entire life. I've had my own challenges in the past with alcohol. This message is not about shaming anyone, but about providing a lifeline that you can grab onto.

With more obesity in the church than in the world, does that mean that more food addicts go to church than not? I doubt it. I think the reason there is more obesity in the church might be twofold. Could it be that gluttony has become the accepted "sin" in church? Second, many gatherings amongst church members revolve around food, and because they don't teach physical stewardship in the church, by and large, the wrong foods are being consumed. It is important to note that a comprehensive review of research on religion, spirituality and health high-lighted that three religious groups show lower weight issues: Amish, Jews, and Buddhists.[10]

It is important for you to understand that there is a divine-human partnership for your health, but perhaps you've never heard it mentioned by your pastor or other church leader. This book speaks volumes about it. I encourage you to read with an open mind and heart. As the Life commercial used to say, "Try it, you'll like it." I will give you suggested resources at the end. Please watch and read them. It is important to educate your-self so you can stay committed to a healthy lifestyle. God has cosmic plans for you. We need you to be in peak health so you can fulfill His purpose in your life! Don't follow but lead your flock with your example. You may just save someone else's life!

---

[10]   https://www.ncbi.nlm.nih.gov/pmc/articles/PMC3671693/ Religion, Spirituality and Health: The Research and Clinical Implications

ENEMY #3–CONFUSION

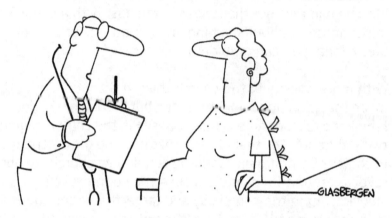

"I want you to follow a healthy lifestyle...
whatever the experts say that is this week."

I love this cartoon.[11] It depicts so well what's happening in our world. Thanks to the Internet and podcasts, there is no lack of health information available to people. If you want a diet that says eat as much chocolate as you want, you will find it. Whatever diet you want to prescribe to, you can probably find someone saying it's beneficial. There is so much confusion around what makes up a healthy diet. Some camps have done a phenomenal job marketing their message, but it is not evidence-based. What does science say?

Neal Barnard, MD, president of the Physician's Committee for Responsible Medicine (www.pcrm.org) summed it up when he said, "Plant-based diets are the nutritional equivalent of quitting smoking."[12] The only diet that science confirms repeat-

---

[11] Randy Glasbergen, 2003

[12] https://journalofethics.ama-assn.org/article/physicians-role-nutri-tion-related-disorders-bystander-leader/2013-04

edly to prevent and reverse the number one killer of both men and women—cardiovascular disease—is a whole-foods plant-based diet. Notice I said "whole-foods", which is the key.

I look to the doctors reversing heart disease, cancer, diabetes, obesity, auto-immune disorders, and more, for my proof. They are reversing these diseases with the power of plants. Michael Greger, MD, who heads up www.nutritionfacts.org, in his book *How Not to Die*[13], shows how you can prevent and reverse the top fifteen killers of Americans with whole-food plant-based diets. What I am suggesting to you is evidence-based with the only potential side effect of having to reduce or eliminate your prescription drugs. I can live with that side effect. How about you?

ENEMY #4—THE MEDICAL PROFESSION

In no way am I condemning the medical profession. Obviously, we need doctors for many things, and most doctors go into the profession with a genuine desire to help people. However, most MDs learn very little nutrition as part of their required curriculum. Only twenty-five percent of medical schools in 2009 required a single course in nutrition, down from thirty-five percent in 2000.[14] A poll showed that only fourteen percent of medical doctors feel confident counseling their patients on proper nutrition.[15] Doctors not knowing what fuel the human body needs, is the equivalent to a car mechanic not knowing what type of fuel your automobile needs. It makes no sense!

Unfortunately, our allopathic medical approach is crisis care. Metaphorically speaking, we place ambulances at the bottom

---

[13] Michael Greger, MD, *How Not to Die, Discover the Foods Scientifically Proven to Prevent and Reverse Disease*, (New York, NY: Flatiron Books, 2015)

[14] https://www.aamc.org/media/25711/download

[15] https://www.ncbi.nlm.nih.gov/pmc/articles/PMC2779722/

of the cliff to treat people when they fall off instead of placing fences at the top to keep them from going over the cliff. My grandfather Daddy Doc was a Medical Doctor in the early 1900's. Back then doctors took a holistic approach and used natural remedies before drugs. I am certain his philosophy had a huge influence on my life and career path, although I barely knew him. It is a pity that doctors are no longer taught how to fuel the human body and how to work with the body instead of shooting the messenger (symptom) with drugs. Michael Greger, MD, says, "The disparity between prevention and mere mitigation of suffering could be a metaphor for modern medicine."[16]

The results of our failed medical system are catastrophic. Global spending for prescription drugs in 2019 was $1.25 trillion and is expected to be $1.59 trillion by 2024. The United States is the top drug user worldwide spending $370 billion annually.[17] A whopping sixty-six percent of Americans take at least one prescription drug daily.[18] The United States ranks forty-sixth in life expectancy in the world.[19] Dr. David S. Ludwig, director of the obesity program at Children's Hospital Boston and one of the authors of a report on obesity and life expectancy said, "Obesity is such that this generation of children could be the first basically in the history of the United States to live less healthful and shorter lives than their parents.»[20] Most doctor visits are for preventable illnesses such as diabetes and heart disease. To top it off, the third leading cause of death

---

[16] Michael Greger, MD, *How Not to Die, Discover the Foods Scientifically Proven to Prevent and Reverse Disease*, (New York, NY: Flatiron Books, 2015)

[17] https://www.statista.com/statistics/280572/medicine-spending-worldwide/

[18] https://hpi.georgetown.edu/rxdrugs/

[19] https://www.worldometers.info/demographics/life-expectancy/

[20] https://www.nytimes.com/2005/03/17/health/childrens-life-expectancy-being-cut-short-by-obesity.html

in America is from iatrogenic causes[21]–the Merriam-Webster dictionary defines iatrogenic as: "induced inadvertently by a physician or surgeon or by medical treatment or diagnostic procedures."[22] Did you catch that? *Medical errors* are the THIRD leading cause of death in America.

Why are you not hearing the information I share with you in this book from the medical associations that should have your back? Or the government? Just follow the money! Dr. Greger explains this in *How Not to Die*, "The American Academy of Family Physicians has a corporate relationship with the Coca Cola Company to support patient education on healthy eating. They have had relationships with Pepsi and McDonalds for some time. Prior to that they had financial ties to cigarette maker Philip Morris. The Academy of Nutrition and Dietetics (formerly American Dietetic Association) publishes sponsored nutrition fact sheets for $20,000 per sheet, paid for by the industries promoting their products. The Academy continues to take millions of dollars from junk food companies, and in exchange they allow these companies to offer educational seminars to teach Registered Dietitians what to recommend to their patients."[23] Do you think this is unbiased information? I don't think so. I won't even go into the relationship between corporate lobbyists and our elected officials and how they are influencing policy makers. The government agencies such as the FDA–Food and Drug Administration–and the CDC–Centers for Disease Control– sadly do not always have your back concerning your health. Until the system changes, expect little change in our health statistics. Thankfully, there are documentaries and books on topics of health that are effecting change little by little (see my lists of recommendations in

---

[21]   https://www.hopkinsmedicine.org/news/media/releases/study_suggests_medical_errors_now_third_leading_cause_of_death_in_the_us

[22]   https://www.merriam-webster.com/dictionary/iatrogenic

[23]   Greger, *How Not to Die* (New York: Flatiron Books, 2015), p. 28

Chapter 6.) For example, if you want to learn how the processed food industry exploits our natural instincts, the emotions we associate with food, and legal loopholes in their pursuit of profit over public health, I recommend the book *Hooked: Food, Free Will, and How the Food Giants Exploit Our Addictions* by Michael Moss[24]. You may be shocked and outraged at what you find out. Please recognize that you and you alone must take control of your health. Don't leave it in your doctor's hands. The responsibility is yours!

ENEMY #5-PRIORITIES

Let's admit it, we don't always have the right priorities in life. It's so easy to let the "not-so-important" things get in the way of the most important things in life. It's the hamster wheel culture we live in that often influences our choices. But there are a lot of things that influence our priorities.

One of my favorite authors is Og Mandino. If you have never read his books, I highly recommend them. I suggest starting with *The Greatest Miracle in the World* and then *The Return of the Ragpicker*. Those books changed my life! He talks about our power to choose in several books. Do you realize we are the only species on the planet that was endowed with the power of choice? All other creatures act based on instinct, but we get to make choices. And our choices determine our lives.

We often choose not to make self-care a priority, especially those of us who are female. We make everyone else a priority above ourselves. I have been teaching people, especially women, to make themselves a priority for years. It's such a hard thing for many women. We take care of the kids, work, our spouse, the dogs, the laundry, whatever, and put ourselves on the bottom of the priority list. Guess what happens when

---

[24]   Moss, *Hooked: Food, Free Will, and How the Food Giants Exploit Our Addictions,* (Random House, 2021)

you are at the bottom of your list? Yep, you never get around to you. It's imperative that we put our own oxygen masks on first. Otherwise, we may not be around for the others we so often prioritize.

Making self-care a priority requires setting healthy boundaries with others and yourself. Of course, we want to be there for other people. We want to help others, it's in our DNA. But unless we are healthy—body, soul and spirit—we will be less effective in helping others. In order to make you a priority, you must put healthy habits on your calendar. You may have to get up an hour earlier to have time to exercise, or pray and meditate, or to do other things that nourish you. You may have to say no to certain activities. Realize that good is the enemy of great. There are many good things you can do, but are they the great things you are called to do? Be willing to say no, so you can say yes to you. You must put your oxygen mask on first!

Here are a few things to consider making self-care a priority:

- **Learn to delegate and ask for help!** Teach your kids to help with chores to free up some of your time. This will require you to give up on perfection, however, because kids will most likely never do things to your standard. For example, I taught my kids to do their laundry when they were twelve years old. My son would inevitably leave his clean clothes in the laundry basket until he wore them, which meant he had wrinkled clothes. I had to let go of being concerned with what others thought of me when they saw him in wrinkled clothes. If he was ok with wearing wrinkled clothes, then that was his choice. Giving kids more responsibility is a win-win. It frees you up to take care of yourself, and it teaches them personal responsibility.

- **Spend less time on social media so you can have time to exercise, read, or spend time with a loved one.** In today's world of instant and constant connection via social media, we lose out on the gift of presence. People often sit looking at their phones while at the dinner table instead of looking loves ones in the eye and having a conversation. It is a sad thing and does not contribute to health. Try taking a social media fast (more on that later) and see how it affects your happiness and health. Be willing to make your dinner table a no-phone zone. Spend time with your kids, grandkids, friends, or family with the phone in the other room to prevent distractions. It's healthy for you and for your loved ones.

- **Limit the time you spend reading or watching the news.** It's a time zapper that only makes you frustrated, sad, or angry. There are rarely good news stories that appear on news sources. Consider getting the Good News Network app for positive news that uplifts instead of the constant negative news. You can read the headlines of news to find out the info you feel you need, unless you are a student and have been instructed to keep up with current events. Eliminating this time and energy zapper will make you healthier, I promise! Try a news fast and see how you feel.

- **Get a set of wireless ear buds and do menial chores while having a conversation on the phone with someone.** While I'm on the phone with loved ones, I grab my dusting mitt and dust, or my broom and sweep, or I fold laundry, or I chop veggies for dinner. If you do this, it will free up more of your time for taking care of yourself. You can also just walk around in your house or yard while you talk on the phone to get more movement in your day.

- **Turn the TV or YouTube off and go to bed.** A good night's sleep is paramount for good health. Your body does a lot of cleansing and repair as you sleep. Set a time that you will be in bed and stick to it. Ideally, you need seven to nine hours of sleep per night for optimal health.

Put you on your priority list and watch your health, happiness, and effectiveness improve. Doing this will benefit you and the ones you love. You will inspire your loved ones to practice self-care through your example.

TIME TO SMILE

Bob and Tom lived in an assisted living facility. They were both in their nineties and had lost their wives. They both loved baseball and had daily talks debating whether there was baseball in Heaven. Tom became sick and it was apparent he wasn't going to make it. Bob asked him to find a way to let him know if there was baseball in Heaven when he got there. Tom passed away and a few days later he appeared to Bob. He said, "Well I have good news and I have bad news. Which do you want first?" Bob replied, "Give me the good news first." Tom said, "Well the good news is there is baseball in Heaven." Bob asked, "What is the bad news?" Tom replied, "You are pitching on Friday."

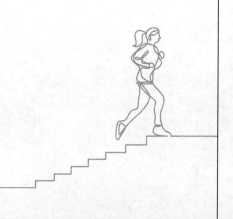

PAY NOW OR PAY LATER

Pay now or pay later. Imagine this picture. You are seventy years old. You have not taken time in your life to exercise. You have not taken time to eat food that is good for your body. The endless cost of the drugs your doctor says you need eats up most of your finances. As you go about your day-to-day life, you grimace at the realization that the quality of your life could have been a lot better had you only cared for yourself better, had you only taken time for your health instead of thinking you were immortal. You justified your actions and even joked about them to others. Now you live in regret and "if only's." Now consider this very different scene. You are seventy years old. Each day you wake up and look out over your peaceful backyard. You and the love of your life take off on a brisk walk, breathing wonderful fresh air and enjoying the surrounding beauty. You return for a healthy breakfast on your deck together. As you go about your day-to-day life, you relish in the abundance you experience thanks to the discipline you exercised during your life. Your past investment of both time and money into your wellness is paying off. You spend no money on drugs, but on the things that keep you healthy. You enjoy the blessings of both health and financial wealth.

Pay now or pay later. The news lately has reported that investing in healthy living now may add up to hundreds of thousands of dollars later in life. I would love to convince you that investing in your wellness increases your wealth and your quality of life. Quality of life is substantially more valuable than any amount of money; however, isn't it exciting to know that taking good care of yourself will pay you financial dividends as well? Sickness is expensive, even if you have good insurance.

As I've emphasized, it is imperative for you to realize that your health is your responsibility. The sooner you get that, the better off you will be. Unfortunately, we live in a culture today that wants relief without responsibility. I believe that is changing. We have reached a point in our history where we can no longer tolerate our bad habits. What is driving the change has a lot to do with how our national health crisis is affecting us financially, both as a country and as individuals. Frankly, we are coming to a place where we simply cannot afford to be sick.

The financial burden of our lack of health is increasingly falling to the consumer (you and I) because employers can no longer afford the skyrocketing health insurance costs. Let's look at some financial implications of this.

In 2019, US healthcare costs were $3.8 trillion, which is the equivalent of $11,582 per person. Health care costs made up nearly eighteen percent of our GDP (Gross Domestic Product) in 2019.[25] Experts estimate that most of those dollars are spent on preventable conditions. For example, cardiovascular disease (still the number one killer in America claiming one-third of American deaths per year) is preventable and eats up $214 billion annually in health care costs. Obesity is another preventable disease and affects nineteen percent of children and forty-two percent of adults. Health care costs related to obesity were $147 billion in 2019. To top it off, over twenty-five percent of adults aged seventeen to twenty-four years old are too overweight to join the military.[26] It's a very sad situation. As I already mentioned, the US spends the most per capita on pharmaceuticals in the world. The average employee's contribution to company provided health insurance has exploded since 2000. There are many people who stay in jobs they hate simply for the health insurance benefit. How sad!

---

[25] https://www.cms.gov/Research-Statistics-Data-and-Systems/
Statistics-Trends-and-Reports/NationalHealthExpendData/
NationalHealthAccountsHistorical

[26] https://www.cdc.gov/chronicdisease/about/costs/index.htm

We correlate the wealth of a country to the health of its people. That is part of the reason we as a nation are in trouble financially. It's time to change this tide. Unfortunately, many people are not willing to change their habits until those habits hit them in the pocketbook. Our country is often that way as well. Bad habits, which have caused poor health, are hitting pocketbooks at alarming rates!

In the western world we have an urgency of excess. Never have such large percentages of the population died from diseases of affluence. Never prior has a financial strain of healthcare distressed every sector of our society, from business to education to government to everyday families.

The answer? Prevention! What does prevention look like? I think it's summed up best by Michael Pollan in his book titled *In Defense of Food*, "Eat real food, not too much, mostly plants."[27] As Dr. Campbell points out so well in his book titled *The China Study*, "We now have a deep and broad range of evidence showing that a whole-food plant-based diet is best for the heart, to prevent cancer, and for diabetes. It's best for every part of our body. The hundreds of well-done research studies all point in the same direction—plant foods!"[28]

Pay now or pay later. Please consider paying now by investing your time and resources in prevention. Not only will it provide you with both quality and quantity of life, but it may be worth tens and even hundreds of thousands of dollars later—a sum that just might exceed your carefully crafted stockpile in your 401K. Investing time and money in your wellness really leads to your wealth, but more importantly, it leads to your health. As John Robbins said, "I'll tell you this: if you want to know what health is worth, ask the person who has lost it."

---

[27]   Michael Pollan, *In Defense of Food, An Eater's Manifesto*, (Penguin Books, 2008)

[28]   T. Colin Campbell, PhD, *The China Study*, (BenBella Books, 2005)

Pay now or pay later. It's really that simple. Do you want to be the seventy-year-old in scenario one lacking quality of life and taking handfuls of costly drugs each day? Or do you want to be the person walking each morning and enjoying an abundant life at age seventy and beyond? *Let's begin with the end in mind. The bottom line: you can invest in your wellness, or you can subsidize your future illness. It is your choice.* I give you a healthy eating and living compass to guide you to your true north of flourishing—body, soul and spirit. I hope you choose to use it to equip you on your journey. It is my sincere desire to see you at destination Peak Health!

WHAT IF?

What if there was one diet and lifestyle that could prevent and reverse the top killer of both men and women in America, cardiovascular disease? What if there was one diet that would prevent and even heal some of the worst cancers? What if there was a lifestyle that helped your children be healthy and live longer? What if there was one diet and lifestyle that eliminated suffering in our world? What if there was a diet that helped you achieve and stay at your optimal weight without feeling deprived? What if there was one diet that prevented and even reversed the top killers in America? What if....? Wouldn't you want to know about it? Wouldn't you tell all your loved ones about it? Wouldn't you be willing to try it? There *is* one diet and lifestyle that can do these things—it is a whole-foods plant-based diet and lifestyle—and I'm committed to help you make it work in your life. I have done it for years and know how to do it easily.

IMAGINE

How much time do you think you spend thinking about and praying for sick people you know? How much time do you think we spend in our churches praying for sick people? How much time do you think we spend worldwide praying for sick people? Now imagine with me for a minute that these people we are praying for who are sick, are instead well. Let's just imagine that sixty percent of them were well and we could free up sixty percent of the countless hours spent praying for sick people who were now well, and instead use all that time to pray for our world. How could that change our world? Just imagine.... Yes, I'm a dreamer. I believe we can get there. One person at a time, drawing a line in the sand and saying, "No more!" No more sickness, no more pain, no more suffering, and no more giving others the responsibility God gave us—personal responsibility for our lives, our health, everything!

I realize that it is often easier to change a person's religion than it is their food. Many foods, especially man-made junk foods, are very addicting. You may be the person who prefers going slow when making changes. If so, I encourage you to focus on adding in the good stuff as opposed to eliminating the bad. The good stuff I recommend adding is Dr. Greger's Daily Dozen which can be followed using the free app you can download on your phone. If you focus on eating the daily dozen, you'll have no room for junk in your belly, I promise. But if you are like me, a draw-the-line-in-the-sand sort of person, then go all out with my recommendations. Say goodbye to foods that don't provide health and hello to foods that help you thrive!

OK let's get going on this plan to optimal health and vitality! I have given you action steps each chapter so you can incorporate something new into each week. I believe in the "inch-by-inch everything is a cinch" philosophy!

ACTION PLAN

1. Spend some time soul searching about the true enemies of your health. Identify your two biggest enemies and journal about why and how they are affecting you. Come up with three ways you will deal with each enemy.

2. Find a counselor or coaching program to help you deal with any emotional issues you feel are causing you to self-sabotage. I recommend you reach out to my friend, Angela Kirtley. She is an Emotion Code Practitioner and someone I highly recommend. You can connect with her via Linked In at https://www.linkedin.com/in/angela-kirtley-ba214244 or email angela.alice510@gmail.com.

3. Write down what you think your priorities are and then look at how you spend your time. Be honest with yourself. If your calendar reflects your priorities, excellent for you! If not, plan to align your life with what you deem most important.

4. Journal about who is impacted by your example and how you would like to be a better influence on them.

5. Share with a buddy your plan to make you a priority and ask them to hold you accountable.

"Those at the top of the mountain didn't fall there."

Marcus Washing

SUMMARY

It is important to understand what tends to undermine your efforts to live a healthy lifestyle so that you can be proactive in eliminating these things. I call these enemies to your health. I've identified five main enemies: you, the flock mentality, confusion, the medical profession, and having the wrong priorities. Unfortunately, we are often our worst enemy. Taking time to figure out how and why you self-sabotage is critical to self-care. The flock mentality can be great for many things but can be a detriment to your health. I encourage you to lead your flock instead of following their bad habits. It's true that we are often the average of the five people we spend the most time with. We tend to adopt the same habits and mindsets of those people. Remember that your example will influence the people you do life with, and you just might save their life, as well as your own. Be willing to be different and uniquely you.

Thanks to a plethora of information available through the internet, people are more confused than ever as to what constitutes a healthy lifestyle. I encourage you to follow the valid science which shows that a whole-food plant-based lifestyle is your best bet for longevity and health. If it can reverse coronary artery disease, Type 2 diabetes, cancer, and more, it can prevent those same diseases and keep you living in vitality. Unfortunately, the medical profession is often the enemy because most doctors are not taught the concept of food as medicine. It's not their fault, it's the system's fault.

Lastly, your priorities dictate how you spend your time. Unfortunately, most people place self-care at the bottom of the list. Follow the advice of the airlines and put your own oxygen mask on first so that you will be there for your loved ones. Self-care pays huge dividends. Remember that your future health starts right now. Be willing to invest now in your wellness so that you can avoid having to pay a huge price later. Disease is expensive. You really are worth it!

God has amazing plans for you and being healthy will allow you to fulfill them. You still have one hundred percent of your life left to live. Make it great by taking care of yourself and getting and staying healthy! You will be so glad you did! Because if you don't take care of your body, where are you going to live? It is the vehicle that carries you around on planet earth. If you want your ride to be smooth and long, take care of your vehicle! It's the only one you have.

CHAPTER 2

NUTRIENTS IN:
FOOD AS MEDICINE

"The doctor of the future will give no
medicine but will instruct their patient in
the care of the human frame, in diet, and
in the cause and prevention of disease."

Thomas Edison

I REMEMBER GROWING up with a human skull in our
house and little jars of natural remedies for mosquito bites,
burns, and the likes, all remnants from my grandfather Daddy
Doc who practiced medicine in the early 1900s. My mother
often continued practicing natural means to deal with illness
throughout my childhood that she had learned from my grandfather. I am convinced that despite Daddy Doc dying while I
was yet young; he influenced my path dramatically.

"Let thy food be thy medicine, and let thy medicine be thy
food.", is a phrase often attributed to Hippocrates, the father of
modern medicine. I have learned the wisdom of the statement
over the years as I have relied heavily on the "food as medicine"
principle as an adult. Before you can truly appreciate how food

is your best medicine, I think you need to understand the role of symptoms in the body.

SYMPTOMS ARE YOUR FRIENDS

Many people view symptoms as enemies, when in fact they are friends. Symptoms are the body's way of telling us that there is something wrong. They are the warning signals of the body, and it is in our best interest to listen to them and not drug them away. We must look at the symptom and determine what it is saying. Symptoms are the body's way of trying to right the wrong so we can return to homeostasis. When we drug the symptom away, we work against the body's defense system. Let me explain.

Medically speaking a symptom is defined as "any indication of disease perceived by the patient."[29] We assume that if the symptom is treated and eradicated, then the disease or illness has been cured.

We view symptoms differently from a natural healing perspective. They are indicators that there is an abnormal condition within the body that is producing a state of "dis-ease." A symptom is the body's effort to eliminate toxins from the body; to return the body to a state of health when stimulated, and to undo any damage done to the body. A symptom is the body's effort at staying alive in the face of wrong-doing, or an invader. Symptoms are the body's attempt to restore health and maintain life. This being the case, it makes sense to deal with the wrong being done instead of eliminating the symptom, or warning signal, through drugs or other means. For example, many times a headache is nothing more than dehydration. Often drinking water will cause the headache to go away, or you may need a chiropractic adjustment.

---

[29] https://medical-dictionary.thefreedictionary.com/symptom

Let's take a fever, for example. The body automatically raises its temperature when confronted with a foreign invader (i.e., virus). The fever is the body's way of killing the invader. Most people immediately try lowering a fever when one appears. What happens when we take Tylenol (or some other toxic drug) to lower the fever? We stop the body's attempt at killing the invader, and the invader gets to live on in the body and create havoc. If, instead of lowering the fever, we go to bed and rest, drink plenty of fluids, and take an enema to ensure the colon's elimination of waste, we encourage the body in its attempt to eliminate the invader. By listening to the symptom and following these natural principles, health returns more quickly, the immune system becomes stronger, we prevent more toxicity by keeping drugs out of the body, and we allow the body to do its job. We have not interfered with the body and its God-given innate intelligence and ability to heal itself.

However, sometimes you need to intervene with a fever, but typically only when you have a compromised immune system brought on by consistent wrong doings. Most adults are fine up to one hundred three degrees Fahrenheit.[30] Prior to it reaching that point, you can try a cool bath which often keeps the temperature from going higher. Most people treat a fever because of how bad it feels to have a higher-than-normal temperature. If you can allow it to run, your body will do its job and kill the invader quicker than if you medicate the symptom away. Please check with your doctor if you spike a high fever as there may be infection present.

Of course, with a fever you need to drink lots of fluids to prevent dehydration. If a child refuses to drink, you can get liquid in them by giving them juice enemas and rubbing them with a wet cloth (the skin will absorb some liquid). I know that juice enemas seem radical, but if your child will not drink during a

---

[30]   https://www.mayoclinic.org/diseases-conditions/fever/symptoms-causes/syc-20352759

fever, you need to get liquid in them, and this is a way to do that. Try giving them popsicles made of pure juice (no sugar) and other healthy liquids that they enjoy.

A fever is just one example of the body doing its job of protecting you and returning you to health. There are many more ways the body works on your behalf—runny nose, cough, skin eruptions, headache, diarrhea, vomiting, etc. I encourage you to listen to your body and try to determine what created the symptom. Then cooperate with the body in eliminating the disease and returning to a state of health and vitality. Instead of being in a hurry to get back to work, why not call in sick, go to bed, and drink plenty of freshly squeezed juice, to give the body more energy for healing? Be patient while your body does its job. Take time to care for your health and therefore reap the benefits in a healthy immune system that can fight off cancer and other diseases that are so prevalent in our society. Again, check with your physician if you have any concern or have symptoms that persist beyond a few days.

Your immune system is designed to take care of you and protect you. When you take care of it, it takes care of you. I have much more faith in my God-given innate immune system than I do any drug or injection. I take care of it by putting nutrients in and keeping toxins out, and so it takes care of me. There is a prevailing attitude in our world (promoted by big pharma) that drugs, vaccines, etc., are somehow more superior than our innate immune system. I simply don't buy it. We were endowed at birth with the most amazing defense system known to man. The problem lies in how we maintain, or more appropriately, fail to maintain our body, including our immune system. The body you are walking around planet Earth in is fearlessly and wonderfully made. It is equipped with everything you need to maintain health and vitality. You may have neglected to maintain your body properly, but you can begin today to take good care of it and rebuild what has been lost. The human body has an amazing capability to heal and restore when treated properly! It can be very forgiving. Take care of it and trust its ability to do its job! The below excerpt says it well.[31]

Excerpt from the book titled *Reclaiming Our Health* by John Robbins:

"Like most people in our society, I grew up believing in the medical myth. I grew up believing that health comes from the doctor, the drugstore, and the hospital. I never suspected that illness might be a messenger, or that our experience of our bodies, whether well or ill, could provide us with self-understanding.

Taken together, factors such as the food we eat, whether and how we exercise, the way we give voice to our feelings, the attitudes we hold, and the quality of the environment in which we live are far more important to the quality of health we experience than even the most sophisticated medical technologies.

In our society, the medical myth has led to an emphasis on intervention instead of prevention that has generated a crisis in health care of epic proportions.

Our medical establishment's fixation on drugs, surgery, and other high-tech interventions at the expense of low-cost preventive approaches is perhaps most evident in its failure to fully appreciate the important role of nutrition in health. The average US physician, in four years of medical school, gets only two hours of course work in nutrition. Only twenty-five percent of the accredited medical schools in the country have a single required course in nutrition. Meanwhile, McDonald's is opening franchises in hospitals!

---

[31]   John Robbins, *Reclaiming Our Health, Exploding the Medical Myth and Embracing the Source of True Healing,* (Tiburon, CA: HJ Kramer, Inc., 1996), p. 2-4

Increasing numbers of us are seeing that we cannot remain passive bystanders to our own health, and then expect the medical system to rescue us. We're seeing how false and destructive is the belief that the more money we spend and the more technology we have, the healthier we will be."

Now that we understand the role of symptoms in health, let's look at what kind of food is the best for the human body.

COLOR YOUR WORLD

One of the major reasons Americans are so sick is because they consume a diet that is very bland, beige, or brown, and less-than-nutritious. We know that the more colorful the food, the more nutritious it is. Consider the MAD (**M**odern **A**merican **D**iet) of meat, potatoes, and bread (brown, beige, or white). Where is the color? Oh yeah, I forgot the salad of iceberg lettuce, eggs, cheese, and croutons—OK right! Iceberg lettuce is mostly white with just a small amount of green.

Adding color to your diet is easy and one of the best things you can do to both prevent disease and heal you when sick. It's best to eat a variety of different colored foods every day. Choose foods with the deepest hues because typically the deeper the color, the more nutritious the food. Eat from each color group to make sure you get a variety of the nutrients that you need each day. Some of the plant's dyes and pigments protect it from sunlight, insects, and disease. For example, the red in tomatoes (the antioxidant called lycopene) protects them from getting sunburned in the sun. Studies have even shown that tomatoes help protect our skin from ultraviolet light as well.[32] The same phytochemicals that protect the plant also

---

[32] https://academic.oup.com/jn/article/131/5/1449/4686953

protect us, so eating lots of brightly colored foods give health protection.[33]

Red foods are excellent at fighting diseases. They contain lycopene, which helps rid the body of free radicals. Free radicals are unstable atoms that wreak havoc in your body. They are a natural by-product of energy metabolism and nature provided the solution to them with antioxidants in plant foods. These seven red foods are excellent disease-fighting fruits and vegetables—cranberries, raspberries, cherries, strawberries, red kidney beans, small red beans, and red apples.

Orange-yellow foods promote heart health. For example, citrus fruits contain carotenoids, which help keep bad (LDL) cholesterol from sticking to artery walls. My mom always told me to eat carrots to maintain good eyesight. Well, she was right as carrots and other orange and yellow foods contain large quantities of beta-carotene that protect against macular degeneration. This color group also lowers cholesterol and contains alpha-carotene, which appears ten times more effective at short-circuiting human cancer cells than beta-carotene.[34]

Dark green vegetables are also very good at fighting disease. Joel Fuhrman, MD, teaches a nutritarian lifestyle that focuses on eating foods that contain the most nutrients per calorie—in other words, nutrient-dense. He is famous for coining the G-BOMBS acronym standing for greens, beans, onions, mushrooms, berries, and seeds. These are the most nutrient dense foods on the planet, and we should eat them every day. He says this on his website about greens: "Leafy greens are the most nutrient-dense of all foods, but unfortunately are only consumed in minuscule amounts in a typical American diet.

---

[33]   https://www.health.harvard.edu/blog/phytonutrients-paint-your-plate-with-the-colors-of-the-rainbow-2019042516501

[34]   https://jamanetwork.com/journals/jamainternalmedicine/fullarticle/226896

We should follow the example of our closest living relatives—chimpanzees and gorillas—who consume tens of pounds of green leaves every day. Leafy greens are also rich in antioxidant pigments called carotenoids, specifically lutein and zeaxanthin, which are the carotenoids known to promote healthy vision. Also, several leafy greens (such as kale) and other green vegetables (such as bok choy, broccoli, and Brussel sprouts) belong to the cruciferous family of vegetables. All vegetables contain protective micronutrients and phytochemicals, but cruciferous vegetables have a unique chemical composition—they contain glucosinolates, and when their cell walls are broken by blending, chopping or chewing, a chemical reaction converts glucosinolates to isothiocyanates (ITCs)—compounds with a variety of potent anti-cancer effects."[35] Research also shows that three servings of spinach per week lowers your risk of macular degeneration by forty-three percent.[36] A study conducted at the Johns Hopkins School of Medicine found the sulforaphane found in broccoli kills helicobacter pylori, the pesky bacteria that causes stomach ulcers and potentially deadly stomach cancers. Sulforaphane can even wipe out strains of helicobacter which are resistant to common antibiotics. They published the findings in the May 28, 2002, issue of the Proceedings of the National Academy of Sciences.[37] The science showing greens are good for human health is impressive. Eat your greens as if your life depends on it, because, well it might.

The **blue and purple** foods (mostly berries) are great at protecting the body from free radical damage. They destroy free radicals before they do any harm to the body. Blue and purple foods are loaded with anthocyanins, which are believed to

---

[35]   https://www.drfuhrman.com/blog/62/
        the-healthiest-anti-cancer-foods-g-bombs

[36]   https://www.scripps.org/
        news_items/3005-eat-your-spinach-save-your-vision

[37]   https://pages.jh.edu/gazette/2002/28may02/28ulcers.html

protect against heart disease by preventing blood clots. Blue and purple foods have top billing on the USDA's power-foods chart (see below). According to James A. Joseph, Ph.D., coauthor of *The Color Code* and chief of the Laboratory of Neuroscience at the USDA Human Nutrition Research Center on Aging at Tufts, blueberries reverse some aspects of aging.[38] We also know them as the brain berry because of their effect on memory. So, eat those blueberries! Wild blueberries contain the most antioxidants as they are smaller and contain more skin, which is where many of the nutrients live. I purchase frozen wild blueberries at Costco and eat one to two cups many nights with a little plant-based milk or yogurt for a nutritious and delicious ice cream substitute.

ORAC, short for Oxygen Radical Absorbance Capacity, is a test tube analysis that measures the total antioxidant power of foods and other chemical substances. High ORAC foods help prevent aging because of their ability to fight free radicals. All plant foods have phytochemicals that are beneficial, and they also contain wonderful fiber that helps keep your colon clean. It is important to take out the trash, and fiber helps your body move it out. Here is a chart showing ORAC values of the top contenders.[39]

---

[38]   Joseph, *The Color Code: A Revolutionary Eating Plan for Optimal Health*, (Hachette Books, 2003)

[39]   https://www.ars.usda.gov/news-events/news/research-news/1999/high-orac-foods-may-slow-aging/

Top-Scoring Fruits & Vegetables

ORAC units per 100 grams (about 3 ½ ounces)

Fruits		Vegetables	
Prunes	5770	Kale	1770
Raisins	2830	Spinach	1260
Blueberries	2400	Brussels sprouts	980
Blackberries	2036	Alfalfa sprouts	930
Strawberries	1540	Brocooli flowers	890
Raspberries	1220	Beets	840
Plums	949	Red bell pepper	710
Oranges	750	Onion	450
Red grapes	739	Corn	400
Cherries	670	Eggplant	390
Kiwi fruit	602		
Grapefruit, pink	483		

MACRO VERSUS MICRONUTRIENTS

The Merriam-Webster Dictionary defines a nutrient as "a substance or ingredient that promotes growth, provides energy, and maintains life."[40] However, there are two types of nutrients—micronutrients and macronutrients. These nutrients serve different purposes in the body, and both are necessary for health.

Macronutrients have caloric value. They provide building blocks for important chemicals in the body needed for overall energy, proper hormonal function, and tissue repair and maintenance. There are three macronutrients—proteins, fats, and carbohydrates. There is much debate in the world today about

---

[40]   https://www.merriam-webster.com/dictionary/nutrient

these three macronutrients and many books are written about them and which kinds serve us best. It can become very confusing for most of us.

Nutrients that do not provide calories are micronutrients. These comprise vitamins, minerals, phytochemicals, and antioxidants. Micronutrients protect molecules from free-radical damage. They help chemical reactions in the body proceed more efficiently and protect cells at the molecular level. Unfortunately, the MAD (**M**odern **A**merican **D**iet) is sorely lacking in micronutrients but abundant in macronutrients. There are thousands of micronutrients with new ones being discovered all the time. You want to eat a micronutrient-rich diet for optimal wellness. Animal products are high in the macronutrients of fat and protein and very low in micronutrients, so they are not an optimal choice for longevity and health.

The bottom line is that we want to choose the macronutrients based on the quality and quantity of micronutrients they provide. For example, potato chips and potatoes are both carbohydrates, but the potato is a better carbohydrate macronutrient to choose because it provides lots of micronutrients that are of an outstanding quality. The potato chip possesses little, if any, micronutrients, and contains "bad" macronutrients in the forms of undesirable fat and processed carbohydrates. The many micronutrients contained in a potato are destroyed in the process to make potato chips.

ANTIOXIDANTS AND PHYTOCHEMICALS

We hear these words a lot, but what do they mean? According to the Concise Medical Dictionary, an antioxidant is any substance that delays the process of oxidation.[41] So what is oxidation? Oxidation is the act or process of combining with oxygen. Oxidation occurs in the normal process of the body converting

---

[41]   Oxford, *Concise Medical Dictionary*, (Oxford University Press: 2010)

food into energy, and in breathing. For example, when you burn wood in the fireplace in the winter, it produces smoke. The smoke represents oxidation, and the resultant ashes are left behind (free radicals) because of the oxidation. Antioxidants go through the body and mop up the ashes, or free radicals, which oxidation leaves behind. You cannot escape oxidation; it is a part of life. God provided the answer to oxidation in antioxidants. Antioxidants come from plant sources only and take care of the oxidation in the body, therefore when you eat plenty of fruits and vegetables, you get plenty of antioxidants to mop up the results of oxidation. When you eat a diet that is lacking in sufficient fruits and vegetables, free radicals take over and leave you with disease.

Phytochemicals are plant chemicals that contain protective, disease-preventing compounds. Phytochemicals are substances that plants naturally produce to protect themselves against viruses, bacteria, and fungi. These compounds play a role in providing the plant's color, their unique taste, and health benefits. They include hundreds of naturally occurring substances that also protect humans, including carotenoids, flavonoids, indoles, isoflavones, capsaicin, and protease inhibitors. A plethora of studies have shown phytochemicals may help protect against some cancers, heart disease, and other chronic health conditions. Phytochemicals like lutein, lycopene and flavonoids are the subject of much research which shows that phytochemicals from foods may help reduce the risk of heart disease and several forms of cancer. Phytochemicals occur in greatest concentration in produce with darker colors or more intense flavor.[42]

I have been asked, "Where do you get your protein?", countless times in the years since I became plant-based in 1976. I'm certain I'd be a millionaire if I just got a dime every time I

---

[42]   https://www.health.harvard.edu/staying-healthy/fill-up-on-phytochemicals

faced that question. Unfortunately, there is an obsession with the macronutrient of protein in America, when in fact, the obsession should be with micronutrients. My response to this question: "Where do you get your phytonutrients and fiber?", or "Where does a cow get its protein?". That leaves people bewildered for sure but in my mind, it exemplifies how very important micronutrients are for the health of the human body. Load up on colorful micronutrients and stop obsessing over carbohydrates and protein. Your body will thank you! Eat the macronutrients which give you the best micronutrient bang for your buck—which are fruits, vegetables, legumes, and whole grains. A great book on this topic is *Proteinaholic* by Garth Davis, MD.[43] If you obsess, like so many, over protein, his book is a must read!

WHY ORGANIC?

What exactly does organic mean? Organic refers to the way we grow and process agricultural products. They base organic food production on a system of farming that maintains and replenishes soil fertility without the use of toxic and persistent pesticides and fertilizers. Organic foods are minimally processed without artificial ingredients, preservatives, or irradiation to maintain the integrity of the food. You can find many studies comparing the nutrient content of organic versus non-organic produce.

I will not go into the research here because it's too extensive. You can do an internet search on organic versus conventional if you want to see the data. I have chosen organic for almost forty years now because I do everything I can to minimize the toxic load to my body. My kids teased me when they were growing up saying my favorite expression was, "It's organic." Whether organic is more nutritious (which many studies show)

---

[43] Garth Davis, MD, *Proteinaholic: How Our Obsession with Meat is Killing Us and What We Can Do About It*, (Harper One, 2015)

or not, it is less toxic since it has not had pesticides and herbicides used on it. Organic produce is guaranteed to be non-GMO, which is important to me and should be important to you too.

I participated in a March Against Monsanto a few years back and was astounded with how many people stopped and asked us what GMO stood for. In case you are unaware of what GMO means, and the risks involved in consuming them, let me give you a short lesson. GMO means "Genetically Modified Organism." Per Zach Bush, MD—a leading expert on the topic of GMO's—a GMO is defined as, "an organism whose genome has been engineered in the laboratory in order to favor the expression of desired physiological traits or the generation of desired biological products."[44] I encourage you to watch his three-hour webinar on the topic found at the link in the footnote. Basically, Monsanto (yes, an agrochemical manufacturer), now Bayer, got in the business of genetically modifying plant seeds to make them Roundup (glyphosate-based herbicide) resistant. In other words, farmers can spray toxic Roundup on the food they grow, and the weeds will die, but the food plant will survive. Do you want the food you eat to be contaminated with a toxic weed killer? I personally don't think it is a good idea, and science is showing the detriments of this practice in agriculture.[45] Dr. Bush goes into extensive detail about the damages caused by the desire to "outsmart mother nature."[46]

GMOs are creating havoc on our planet as well as our health. That is why I urge you to choose non-GMO products. However, be aware that the "non-GMO Verified" label does not mean the product is non-toxic. Many items contain this label, and although it is important to eat non-GMO food as I've alluded to,

---

[44] Bush, *GMO's: Engineering the Nature Out of Humanity*, https://zach-bushmd.com/gmo-1/

[45] http://responsibletechnology.org/docs/gmos-are-not-safe.pdf

[46] https://zachbushmd.com/gmo-2/

the label does not guarantee the lack of toxic pesticides and herbicides. For example, many grains and legumes—such as oats, wheat, and lentils—are typically not genetically modified, but farmers spray glyphosate (the herbicide in Roundup) on these crops a couple of weeks prior to harvest as a desiccant (drying agent). Therefore, you should always choose organic for grains and legumes—non-GMO verified makes little difference in these cases as they were sprayed with glyphosate close to harvesting.[47] Buying certified organic products is the only way to know you aren't getting a dose of Roundup in your food. You can also talk to local farmers to see if they use toxic pesticides and herbicides. Of course, growing what you can yourself is a great way to feel confident in your food! Also, please note that there is a new certification underway that goes beyond non-GMO Verified—it's called Glyphosate-Residue Free.[48] I'm excited for that label to become mainstream!

Many raise the concern with me regarding the price of organic versus non-organic. My feeling is that it's an investment in both me and my family's health, and our environment. If you absolutely cannot buy organic because of price or availability, then make sure and wash your produce very well to remove as much of the chemicals and pesticides as possible. You can find good, non-toxic cleaners at health food stores or you can make your own by mixing one cup of vinegar with four cups of water in a spray bottle, and then add one tablespoon of lemon juice. Spray your produce liberally in a colander in your sink and allow it to sit two to five minutes, then rinse well. Also, you can order things like organic beans and grains in bulk online for a huge discount.

Here are my recommendations on buying organic:

---

[47]   https://www.cornucopia.org/2017/10/
glyphosate-use-desiccant-doubles-human-contamination/

[48]   https://detoxproject.org/certification/glyphosate-residue-free/
certified-products/

1. Buy organic if you can afford it because it is better for the environment and your body.

2. Print out the Dirty Dozen list every year from the Environmental Working Group (www.EWG.org) and try to always buy organic of the items on this list, if possible.

3. Grow your own garden so you can control what goes on it. There are many gardening books you can pick up at your local library. I recommend growing in an aeroponics environment using Tower Gardens™ (you can learn more about them at www.TowerofEden.com). They eliminate the dirt, weeding, and use 10% of the water and land of traditional gardening.

4. Checkout www.OrganicConsumers.org for many great resources.

5. Purchase from a local farmer's market for the freshest produce. Ask the people questions about their growing methods. Many times, you will find they use sustainable practices even if they don't grow certified organic produce. You can typically find many pesticide-free and organic growers at farmer's markets. And it's always great to support local growers.

6. If you can't get or afford organic, eat the produce anyway. Studies showing the effectiveness of fruits and vegetables in human health were done with conventional produce most of the time. They show substantial benefit from eating fruits and vegetables, regardless of whether they grow it organically. Just remember to wash non-organic produce well as I mentioned above.

SATISFY YOUR SWEET TOOTH WITH FRUIT

The 2010 Global Burden of Disease Study, which involved five hundred researchers, determined the leading cause of both death and disability in the US, followed by smoking, was not eating enough fruit.[49] Fruit and other carbohydrates have gotten a bad rap in today's world with fad diets such as keto and paleo. Unfortunately, there is no scientific data showing fruit is bad for human health. Quite the contrary. Fruit is an ideal food and is the perfect food to satisfy our natural sweet tooth. I call it nature's candy. It is full of natural sugars that give us energy, lots of micronutrients, and beneficial fiber. Fruit is safe for diabetics (read *Dr. Neal Barnard's Program for Reversing Diabetes*[50]) in its natural, complete state—best eaten whole instead of in juice form. Fruit is the easiest food to digest, and most fruits provide a significant source of hydration because they are juicy. However, if you need to lose weight, steer clear of dried fruit such as raisins and dates as the calories and sugars are more concentrated in dried fruit.

Fruit is one of the best "fast foods" on the planet. It is so easy to grab a piece of fruit when rushing out the door. Fruit is also a great quick energy source. Fruit is technically anything with a seed within, so things we typically think of as vegetables such as peppers, tomatoes, and avocados, are fruit. Berries give the best overall nutrition per calorie (as shown earlier in the ORAC chart). Studies have shown tart cherries to reduce inflammation and help with gout.[51] Goji berries contain the highest concentration of melatonin and help people with

---

[49]   https://nutritionfacts.org/topics/fruit/

[50]   Neal Barnard, MD, *Dr. Neal Barnard's Program for Reversing Diabetes: The Scientifically Proven System for Reversing Diabetes Without Drugs*, (Rodale Books, 2018)

[51]   https://nutritionreview.org/2015/04/new-study-tart-cherries-reduce-uric-acid-levels-gout-and-c-reactive-protein-inflammation/

macular degeneration.[52] [53] [54] Research has shown berries to protect against cancer, boost your immune system, guard the liver and brain, and protect against cardiovascular disease. The darker the berry or fruit, the more nutritious. For a more detailed explanation on the tremendous benefits of fruit, I highly recommend the book *How Not to Die* by Michael Greger, MD.

Satisfy your sweet tooth with fruit and help prevent all kinds of maladies and heal your body! Fruits help cleanse the body. Don't buy into the anti-fruit propaganda. It's not based on science.

VEGETABLES TO THE RESCUE

One cannot overstate the value of vegetables in the prevention and treatment of disease. This is the one thing that most diets promoted today agree on—eat lots of vegetables, especially leafy greens. The serving recommendations I list here are based on Dr. Greger's Daily Dozen.[55]

Leafy green vegetables are the healthiest food on the planet as they provide the most nutrition per calorie. Science shows that daily consumption of leafy greens prolongs life. They give us the strongest protection against chronic disease, including cancer. They are so valuable that General George Washington issued a general order in 1777 that troops should forage for wild greens around their camps "as these vegetables are very

---

[52]   https://nutritionfacts.org/topics/goji-berries/

[53]   https://pubmed.ncbi.nlm.nih.gov/21169874/

[54]   https://www.webrn-maculardegeneration.com/goji-berries-benefits.html

[55]   https://nutritionfacts.org/topics/daily-dozen/

conducive to health and tend to prevent all putrid disorders."[56] Green vegetables are also a wonderful source of bioavailable calcium and will contribute to strong bones (more about that in the section on dairy). Green leafy vegetables include all lettuces, spinach, and greens such as kale and collard greens. Sadly, only four percent of Americans eat the recommended two servings per day. A serving is one cup of raw or one-half cup of cooked. Harvard University found a twenty per-cent reduction in risk for both heart attacks and strokes for every additional serving of greens you eat per day. So, Popeye was right, eat your greens! You can eat unlimited green veg-etables but aim for at least two servings per day. The more, the better![57]

Cruciferous vegetables are also powerhouses and are part of a healthy diet. The name cruciferous comes from the Latin word for crucifix because the blossoms of these plants look like a cross. Cruciferous veggies include broccoli, cauliflower, bok choy, arugula, kale, cabbage, turnips, radishes, and Brussel sprouts. As you can see, some cruciferous veggies also fit in the leafy green category. That means if you eat kale as one of your servings of green leafy veggies, it doesn't also count as a cruciferous vegetable serving. Cruciferous vegetables are best known for their anti-cancer effect on the body, but the ben-efits of this class of vegetables are endless. They help detox the body, prevent DNA damage, defend against pathogens and pollutants, and help protect your brain and vision. Eat as many as you want, but at least one serving per day. I roast two of my favorite things to eat: broccoli and cauliflower. You can also throw spinach or kale in a smoothie for a simple way to get

---

[56] Greger, Michael. *How Not to Die, Discover the Foods Scientifically Proven to Prevent and Reverse Disease*, (New York, NY: Flatiron Books), p. 311

[57] https://www.drfuhrman.com/blog/62/
the-healthiest-anti-cancer-foods-g-bombs

it in the raw form daily, especially for kids. They won't even know it's there!

You will want to eat a variety of other vegetables every day besides your leafy greens and cruciferous veggies, at least an additional two servings. See the Daily Dozen app for suggestions!

Remember, as with fruits, the darker the color, the better for your health. It is best to eat as many in their complete form as possible with their skin. The skin has many nutrients. For example, the skin of the sweet potato has significantly more of the antioxidant power as the inner flesh on a per weight basis.[58] That puts the sweet potato skin on the same level as blueberries, antioxidant-wise. You want diversity in your vegetable intake because different colors have different effects on the body as we learned previously. Many people eat the same thing over and over, but it's always best to eat a variety of colorful fruits and vegetables daily.

Fruits and vegetables are so important that they literally could save your life. A union of concerned scientists estimates that if the nation increased its consumption of fruits and veggies to meet the dietary guidelines of seven to twelve servings per day, that it could save over one hundred thousand people per year.[59] Don't you want to get that kind of protection? Eat your fruits and veggies to prevent disease and heal your body. The more, the better!

---

[58]   https://www.livestrong.com/
article/534200-what-nutrients-are-in-the-skins-of-sweet-potatoes/

[59]   https://www.ucsusa.org/about/news/
extra-daily-serving-fruits-or-vegetables

LEGUMES—THE DIETARY FOUNTAIN OF YOUTH

Beans, beans, the musical fruit, the more you eat, the more you toot. Beans, beans, they're good for your heart, the more you eat, the more you fart. These two little rhymes we have all heard remind of us of the number one reason many people shy away from eating beans—because they cause gas. Hippocrates said, "Passing gas is necessary to well-being."[60] As Michael Greger, MD says, "You can pass gas, or you can pass on." Which will it be? But seriously, beans are one of the most beneficial foods for your body. Many studies have found an association between bean consumption and longevity.[61] (Now I know why my father-in-law is still alive and well at ninety-three! He eats lots of beans, and to boot, he eats lots of greens too! Beans and greens are a powerful duo for sure!)

The resistant starch in beans causes the gas, but it also promotes satiety, lowers glucose levels, increases fat burn, promotes bowel regularity, and reduces fat storage after a meal. Beans are also loaded with fiber, which helps your body in many of the same ways. It lowers cholesterol by binding it for removal from the body. Fiber fills up your stomach and signals your brain that you are full. We need a fiber-rich diet and beans are such a dominant source. It's hard to experience constipation on a bean-rich diet thanks to the great fiber and resistant starch content.

Besides lowering cholesterol, beans also lower blood pressure, give you a slimmer waist, regulate blood sugar and insulin levels[62], reduce your risk of stroke, depression, and colon can-

---

[60]   Greger, Michael. *How Not to Die, Discover the Foods Scientifically Proven to Prevent and Reverse Disease*, (New York, NY: Flatiron Books), p. 287

[61]   https://nutritionfacts.org/video/increased-lifespan-from-beans/

[62]   https://www.drfuhrman.com/blog/95/clinical-study-confirms-that-beans-are-the-preferred-starch-source-for-diabetics

cer.[63][64] Science shows soybeans prevent and improve breast cancer survival.[65] My gosh, with these benefits, why would you not eat beans? The bean family includes lentils, pintos, black beans, garbanzos, black-eyed peas, etc.

I'm simply highlighting the research on these foods. For a more detailed look at all the research on how any of these items relate to health, again I point you to *How Not to Die* by Michael Greger, MD, or go to www.NutritionFacts.org.

What I have found is that the more you eat beans, the less gas you will get as your body adjusts to the resistant starch. I'm not saying you won't have any, but you will find it more manageable. I have also found that canned or powdered beans give more gas than pre-soaked beans cooked in a pressure cooker. I have an Instant Pot which is fabulous for cooking dried beans quickly. I recommend soaking the beans overnight in water or my preferred method of putting dried beans in the Instant Pot with plenty of water. Turn it on manual for four minutes of high-pressure cooking, then allow it to sit for ten minutes. At this point you can drain and rinse the beans and return them to the pot with onions, garlic, and seasonings. Put them on the "bean" mode, which is thirty minutes. You will have the most delightfully tender beans cooked this way, and they will give you less gas. Eat at least three servings of beans every day for longevity and health. A serving is one-fourth cup of hummus or bean dip, one-half cup cooked beans, lentils, tofu or tempeh, or one cup of fresh peas.

---

63 https://chopra.com/articles/5-ways-beans-boost-your-heart-health

64 https://www.medicalnewstoday.com/articles/320192#benefits

65 https://foodrevolution.org/blog/soy-facts-is-soy-healthy/

WHOLE GRAINS – YOU'RE WELCOME

Yes, I'm suggesting you eat whole grains. You are welcome! Notice I said 'whole' which is not the processed grains that many people eat. Whole grains such as whole wheat, brown rice, quinoa, millet, buckwheat, amaranth, oats and corn are all excellent food for humans and contribute to longevity. Unfortunately, the anti-carb camp has demonized a food group that is a predominant food amongst the people who live the longest disability-free, as portrayed in the book by Dan Buettner titled *The Blue Zones: 9 Lessons for Living Longer from the People Who've Lived the Longest*. Not only do whole grains lead to longevity, but they also reduce your risk of heart disease, type two diabetes, obesity, and stroke. They also reduce inflammation in the body.[66]

Concerning longevity, the famous Harvard Nurses Study and Health Professionals Follow-up Study accumulated three million person-years of data. Their 2015 analysis showed that people who eat more whole grains live significantly longer lives, independent of other dietary and lifestyle factors.[67]

Don't buy into the anti-carb movement that benefits from incredible marketing. Carbohydrates are what your body uses for energy. They are good for you. The problem we have gotten into is that there are so many junk food products on the market that are carbohydrates; however, they are the bad carbs. As I mentioned earlier, choose your macronutrients based on how many micronutrients they contain. For example, white bread contains the macronutrient of carbohydrate, but it has virtually no micronutrients at that point after being processed so heavily. But if you take whole wheat, it is full of carbohydrates, but they are good carbs. Whole wheat is full of beneficial

---

[66] https://draxe.com/nutrition/whole-grains/

[67] https://www.hsph.harvard.edu/news/press-releases/
more-whole-grains-linked-with-lower-mortality-risk/

micronutrients and fiber. Carbs are not bad for you if they are the good carbs which contain wonderful micronutrients and fiber. Whole grains are a good carb and necessary for health and longevity. They also keep your bowels moving, which is so very important for your health. Remember, you want to take out the garbage and fiber does that for you!

Eat at least three servings per day of whole grains to increase your lifespan and quality of health. A serving is one-half cup of hot cereal (such as oatmeal), cooked grains (such as brown rice or quinoa), pasta, or corn kernels. Other serving sizes are one whole grain tortilla or slice of bread, one-half of a bagel or English muffin, or three cups of popcorn. It is important to read labels to see if the product is whole grain or not. Many breads claim that they are whole wheat but really are not. You can tell by looking at bread if it is whole or not. Whole-grain breads are typically more dense and darker. I prefer Ezekiel sprouted breads and my husband likes Dave's Killer bread. We get organic whole wheat tortillas at Costco. Oatmeal is a great way to start the day, and you can even make overnight oats to have them ready in the morning. Add a bunch of berries for a micronutrient-rich start to your day. Again, you are welcome!

WHAT ABOUT NUTS AND SEEDS?

Nuts and seeds are a part of a healthy whole-food plant-based diet. However, they are very calorie dense, so you need to watch how many you eat. I take the advice of Dr. Greger and suggest one tablespoon of ground flaxseeds or chia seeds daily, and one-fourth cup of raw walnuts or other nuts (see the Daily Dozen app). There is much debate in the plant-based community over whether to include nuts and seeds in your diet. Based on scientific evidence, I think it is important to include some of them for optimal health. Your brain needs fat and there are certain vitamins (A, D, E, and K)[68] that are fat-soluble, meaning they need fat for absorption by the body. For example, leafy greens have a lot of fat-soluble nutrients, so it is always a good idea to add some nuts, seeds, or avocado to your salad to boost nutrient absorption.[69]

Nuts have plant sterols which are compounds that help block your body from absorbing cholesterol. While plant sterols help lower LDL cholesterol (the bad kind), they don't appear to affect your levels of HDL cholesterol (the good kind) or tri-glycerides. Certain nuts and seeds are high in omega-3 essential fatty acids which are beneficial for heart and brain health. The highest concentration of EFA's in the plant kingdom is found mainly in walnuts, flaxseeds, and chia seeds.[70] "Essential" means you must get them from food, your body does not make them.

Nuts and seeds also contain L-arginine, an amino acid that is an essential protein building block in your body. L-arginine helps make artery walls more flexible, aids in wound healing, aids the kidneys in removing waste products from the body, and helps maintain immune and hormone function in the body. Other plant-based sources of L-arginine include legumes and whole grains.[71]

Another beneficial part of nuts and seeds is fiber. I've already discussed the benefits of a fiber-rich diet. The fiber in nuts and

---

[68]   https://findgoodhealth.org/
list-of-vitamins-and-supplements-water-fat-soluble/

[69]   *Forgo Fat-Free Dressings?*, https://nutritionfacts.org/video/
forego-fat-free-dressings/

[70]   *Essential Fatty Acids from Plant Foods*, https://www.downtoearth.org/
health/nutrition/essential-fatty-acids-plant-foods

[71]   *L-Arginine Foods: 12 Highest Sources*, https://www.superfoodly.
com/l-arginine-foods/

seeds may explain why they are good at lowering the bad LDL cholesterol in the body.

CULTURED VEGETABLES FOR YOUR GUT

Vegetables are nature's most perfect food. They are full of vitamins, minerals, phytochemicals, and enzymes. They also help to alkalinize the body. Unfortunately, many people's digestive systems are too weak or compromised to digest vegetables, despite their abundant enzymes, due to all the cellulose (fiber) they contain. A major cause of poor digestion is that our adrenal and thyroid glands are poorly nourished and taxed by toxins and stress. As a result, many people experience gas and bloating when they eat a lot of vegetables. I recommend a good digestive enzyme supplement to help the body break down the cellulose in vegetables. Fermenting your vegetables is another brilliant solution.

Traditionally fermenting foods is a great way to boost your nutrition and help your digestive system. Fermented foods such as sauerkraut, cultured vegetables, live pickles, and Kimchi are excellent sources of nutrients, enzymes, and probiotics. Raw cultured vegetables have been around for centuries and have reemerged in the last twenty years as a wonderful addition to a healthy diet. Eating one-half cup to a cup of raw cultured vegetables with your meals will help digest the food you eat. Consuming them daily will also help repair a compromised digestive system.

The website http://www.rejuvenative.com/ (where you can buy cultured veggies if you don't want to make them yourself) explains the science of fermentation as: «Many different microorganisms, present in nature, are found in all vegetables. In cabbage, these organisms mostly stay on the surface of the leaf. But if cabbage leaves are ground up, this exposes the inner part of the leaf for bacterial colonization. Left at room temperature, the ground-up cabbage will soon be permeated with *leuconostoc mesenteroides*, which lower the pH to a more acidic environment. In this environment, the *lactobacillus acidophilus* and *lactobacillus plantarum* thrive. They rapidly produce enzymes which convert sugars and starches into more lactic and acetic acid. These acids now act as preservatives, discouraging harmful bacteria and mold. After six days of fermentation, the conversion process peaks, and the microflora dwindle. Under refrigeration, the conversion process continues more slowly. Thus, raw cultured vegetables keep their nutrition, flavor, and health benefits."[72]

I don't recommend most varieties of sauerkraut you get in the store. They are often high in sodium and low in probiotics. You can find some raw brands like Rejuvenative—mentioned above—in stores, especially health food stores. You will always find these brands in the refrigerated section of the store. You can find an organic brand at Costco as well. I recommend making your own if you can, as they are very easy to make and are much less expensive.

Here is the recipe I recommend:

- 1 large or 3 smaller heads of purple or green cabbage
- several carrots or a bunch of kale
- 1 beet
- 1 large chunk of ginger, and/or several garlic cloves, optional
- 1-3 tablespoons of Himalayan or Celtic Salt

Remove several of the outer leaves of the cabbage to use in the tops of the jars. Set aside. To make this recipe, shred or thinly slice the veggies and add to a large bowl with the salt. Remove several cups of the vegetables and add them to a

---

72   *A Guide to Raw Cultured Vegetables*, https://www.rejuvenative. com/a-guide-to-raw-cultured-vegetables/

blender. Add several cups of pure water and blend to make a thick brine. Add this brine back to the bowl and mix well. Press the veggies down into quart-sized glass jars and fill to almost full. Leave a half-inch for the veggies to expand. Take a large cabbage leaf and roll and place on top of the veggies. Seal the jars. Place the jars on a counter in room temperature of at least 70 degrees. Allow to sit for up to a week to allow for fermentation. Morning and night turn the jars over to allow the brine to cover all the veggies. Return them to their upright position. You will see the brine expand during the week as the vegetables ferment. Starting on the third day, open the jar and taste a bite to make sure it has a nice sour taste. Once the veggies have soured sufficiently, place the jars in the refrigerator to slow the fermentation process. They should last for many months in the refrigerator. They will continue to ferment but very slowly due to the low temperature.

The benefits of consuming cultured vegetables include improved digestion (because of the microbes they include that introduce beneficial bacteria to the gut), improved immunity (thanks to the probiotics provided), detoxification (the bacteria in them help detoxify your body and remove heavy metals), better energy (they help your body function more efficiently), improved mental health (there is a gut/brain connection), and stronger overall health (good health begins in the gut).[73]

Enjoy cultured vegetables daily to restore your gut microflora. Make it a daily habit and be patient with restoring your gut. If you don't like the taste of these "sour" foods, eat them anyway because they can be powerful medicine for your body. I don't care for the taste of cultured veggies, but I eat them because they are good for me. I sometimes add my tablespoon of ground flaxseeds to my cultured veggies, which tones down the sour taste and makes them more palatable for me. Mixing them with other foods you are eating can also tone the sour down.

---

[73]   https://www.superfoodevolution.com/cultured-vegetables.html

Kids often like them, which is great! Remember that healing takes time. Be patient with the process. You are worth it.

ALKALINIZE YOUR BODY WITH FOOD

Another important aspect of good nutrition is eating the proper ratio of acid and alkaline foods. Foods either leave an alkaline ash in the body or an acid ash. The ash is the residue left behind by the food. If it is acidic, the body must neutralize it to keep the blood from becoming too acidic. Blood PH must be an alkaline balance of around 7.35-7.45. The pH scale ranges from zero to fourteen. The level of seven is considered neutral. Below seven is acidic and above seven is alkaline.

The body protects the blood at all costs. The cells of the body that are in a healthy state are alkaline. When a body is diseased, it will be more acidic, and the more acidic the cells of the body become, the sicker the body is, and the worse you feel. Our body produces acid as a normal by-product of metabolism. It does not produce alkaline; therefore, we must depend on alkaline foods in order to replenish the body's alkalinity. The more alkaline our cells become, the more energy we have. Cancer survives in an acid environment.[74]

The optimal diet comprises seventy to eighty percent alkaline foods and only twenty to thirty percent acid foods.[75] Interestingly, that is the exact ratio of foods found in nature. Unfortunately, the average American diet comprises just the opposite—only twenty to thirty percent alkaline foods and seventy to eighty percent acidic foods. I have included a chart of acid and alkaline foods in Chapter 6—Your Thrival Guide.

---

[74]   https://www.alternative-cancer-care.com/acid-alkaline-ph-and-cancer.html

[75]   Joel Robbins, DC, ND, *Health Through Nutrition*, https://www.dajonline.net/Health/Health_through_Nutrition/

ACTION PLAN

1. **Power Up Your Produce**–This is the number one thing you can do to improve your health! Eat two to four servings of raw fruits and/or vegetables with every meal to add vital enzymes and nutrients to your diet. A serving is as follows:

   - One medium-sized fruit (i.e., apple, orange, banana, pear)
   - 1/2 cup of raw or frozen fruits or vegetables
   - 3/4 cup (6 oz.) of one hundred percent fruit or vegetable juice, freshly made
   - 1/2 cup cut-up fruit
   - 1 cup of raw, leafy vegetables (i.e., lettuce, spinach)
   - 1/4 cup dried fruit (i.e., raisins, apricots, mango – organic, unsulfured only)

2. **Download Dr. Greger's Daily Dozen app** on your phone (it's free) and begin to familiarize yourself with the daily dozen items. Click on each item and watch at least one video relating to that item.

3. Have fun and realize that **nothing tastes as good as fit and healthy feel!**

4. Take a trip to the produce department of your grocery store and find the most colorful produce. Buy two items you have never tried before.

"The science is clear. The results are unmistakable. Change your diet and dramatically reduce your risk of cancer, heart disease, diabetes and obesity. By any measure, America's health is failing. We spend far more, per capita, on health care than any other society in the world, and yet two-thirds of Americans are overweight, and more than fifteen million Americans have diabetes. We fall prey to heart disease as often as we did thirty years ago. The War on Cancer, launched in the 1970's, has been a miserable failure. Half of all Americans have a health problem that requires taking a prescription drug every week, and more than one hundred million Americans have high cholesterol. To make matters worse, we are leading our youth down a path of disease earlier and earlier in their lives. One-third of the children in this country are overweight or at risk of becoming overweight. Our kids are increasingly falling prey to a form of diabetes that used to be seen only in adults, and children now take more prescription drugs than ever before. These issues all come down to three things: breakfast, lunch and dinner."

T. Colin Campbell, PhD in The China Study

CHAPTER 3

READY, SET, RESTORE

"I don't care how old I live! I just want to be living while I am living!"

Jack LaLanne on his 90th birthday

FASTING CAN SAVE YOUR LIFE

I LOVE THIS quote from Jack LaLanne on his ninetieth birthday.[76] I translate it to: "I want to live all the years I'm alive." How about you? Don't you want to live all the years you are alive? Would you like to die young late in life? Okay, I know you need a minute to think about that one. I'm sure when you realize what I just asked you, your answer will be a resounding YES! All of us deep down want to live a long, healthy life. Where the rubber meets the road is when you must decide if you will do what it takes to make that wish a reality. Fasting is a powerful way to help you die young late in life and live all the years you are alive!

The definition of restore from <u>dictionary.com</u> is: to bring back to or put back into a former condition; repair or renovate, so

---

[76] https://quotefancy.com/jack-lalanne-quotes

as to return it to its original condition.[77] This chapter is about using the power of fasting as a tool to restore the body to the state of homeostasis, or health. We live in a world of dietary excess where we feast every day, often three times per day. While feasting is good on holidays and special occasions, it is not good daily. I do not know of any more effective tool than fasting for helping you to step out of the dietary excess game and turbocharge your healing process. There are many types of fasts which can help you. Fasting is not only beneficial from a physical standpoint, but also is a great tool to become more spiritually healthy.

JUICE FASTING

Thanks to the incredible documentary titled *Fat, Sick and Nearly Dead*, juicing for health and well-being has had a resurgence in the public awareness. As a Naturopath and health coach, I have learned about and tried a variety of fasts and health regimes. In the form of a juice fast, juicing for health is one of the safest and most impactful methods I have seen work on myself and my clients. There are many healing therapies that incorporate juicing for health, such as the Gerson Therapy (www.gerson.org) which heals cancer and other degenerative diseases. It is a simple concept, but one that requires effort. For disease-specific juice recipes, I recommend picking up a copy of Dr. Norman Walker's classic book titled *Fresh Vegetable and Fruit Juices*.[78]

BENEFITS OF DAILY JUICING FOR HEALTH:

- **Live nutrition from raw, living plant foods.** Juicing provides the best vitamin/mineral supplement you can get! Remember that life begets life! Unfortunately, most

---

[77]   https://www.dictionary.com/browse/restore

[78]   Norman Walker, D.Sc., *Fresh Vegetable and Fruit Juices, What's Missing in Your Body?*, (Norwalk Press, rev. 1978)

people are operating from a nutritional deficit because of less-than-ideal diets. Consistent juicing eliminates the deficit and floods your body with healing nutrients and enzymes. Enzymes are the life force of food. They are complex substances which enable you to digest food and absorb it into your bloodstream. The action and activity of every atom in your body intimately involves enzymes, hence they are catalysts. Where there is life, there are enzymes. Live food begets life!

- **Easy assimilation of nutrients.** Most people who have consumed a less-than-ideal diet over the years have degenerated their digestive system and do not digest, absorb, and process the nutrients in their food efficiently. Juicing bypasses this issue as the juicing process breaks the food down into tiny particles that require very little digestive effort. The juice and nutrients go into the gut for absorption. That is why it is always ideal to drink juice on an empty stomach and wait at least twenty to thirty minutes until you eat food. When you drink fresh-squeezed juice, you get up to ninety-five percent of the nutrients and they are available quickly to your cells. Juicing provides healing nutrients of raw fruits and vegetables in their whole, complete and living form.

- **Conservation of energy.** It requires a lot of the body's energy to digest food. The heavier the food, the more energy it takes. For example, it takes much more energy to digest meat than it does potatoes and more energy to digest potatoes than fruit. Since juices involve very little digestion, it requires almost no energy. This reserves the body's energy for other tasks, such as healing.

- **Detoxification.** Consuming daily fresh vegetable and fruit juices helps your body cleanse and detox. Getting the toxins out of your body is paramount to healing. Today's world exposes us to many toxins from the air, water, cleaning and personal care products, and our food. Eating organic minimizes your toxic load, but no matter how "clean" your life is, it's impossible to escape toxins in the world. Juicing helps the body's ability to rid it of toxins (more on detoxification below).

- **Fruit juices are cleansers. Vegetable juices are nourishers.** For optimal results, drink at least sixteen ounces per day, more if you are sick. The more you drink, the quicker you will experience results.

- **Gets nutrients in and toxins out!** Both requirements for health and healing are met through juicing. Win-win!

BENEFITS OF A JUICE FAST:

- A means of providing high concentrations of healing nutrients in a form that requires very little digestion and assimilation of energy.

- Allows the digestive system to rest and rebuild.

- Juicing does away with indigestion, a lack of proper digestion.

- Juicing allows the body to both detoxify and heal.

- A one-month juice diet is the equivalent of five to six months on a raw fruit and vegetable diet.

INSTRUCTIONS FOR AN EFFICIENT JUICE FAST:

- Juice must be freshly made using a high-quality juicer such as a Green Star. For cancer patients, a Norwalk juicer is recommended.

- Juice only organic produce. Otherwise, you are getting a toxic cocktail!

- Sip juice slowly—consume between ½ gallon and 1 gallon daily.

- If the body loses its appetite, listen to it. It desires a rest and probably wants to do some cleansing. Drink only distilled water and very diluted (fifty percent) juice. Do not continue for more than two days on this program without the supervision of a health provider, as it more closely resembles a water fast.

- If something is desired to chew, eat melons. An occasional piece of raw, juicy fruit is acceptable, but no more than once a day.

- Do not drink after 8:30 PM.

- Drink purified water as desired.

- Exercise twice daily as it increases the efficiency of the diet, but don't overdo it. Lighter exercise is preferred, such as walking.

- Take one or two fifteen-to-thirty-minute catnaps daily. Get at least nine hours sleep at night if possible. Your body is doing some major cleansing and healing and needs rest!

- It is essential to have at least one bowel movement daily to aid in the removal of toxins from the body. To ensure this, take one tablespoon of ground flaxseeds or chia seeds in one of your juices to get the fiber needed. To help your colon continue moving, drink Traditional Medicinal Smooth Move tea nightly. If you have not had a bowel movement that day, then take a clear water enema before bedtime.

- Take a good quality probiotic two times daily. Take on an empty stomach.

PREPARING FOR THE JUICE FAST (3 DAYS PRIOR):

- Decrease your consumption of food and eat your last meal by six PM.

- Eat only fresh fruit for breakfast.

- Your last meal the night before your fast should be all raw fruits and veggies.

BREAKING THE JUICE FAST:

- Eat only fruits for the first two days after completing the juice diet. The third day you may introduce raw veggies. Continue with only raw for another day. You may add cooked food on the fourth day after the juice diet, or sooner if you did a shorter fast.

- Breaking the juice diet properly is as important as the diet itself. If you break this type of regime improperly, you can undo some of the good that was accomplished.

JUICE RECIPES (USE ALL ORGANIC PRODUCE)

General Nourishing Daily Juice:

- 3-4 carrots
- 1 beet
- 1 cucumber
- ½ to 1-inch piece of ginger
- 1 granny smith apple

- 4 stalks celery
- 1 bunch of parsley

Juice for Allergies:

- 10 ounces carrot juice
- 3 ounces celery juice
- 3 ounces cucumber juice

Juice for Eczema:

- 16 ounces of celery juice OR
- 7 ounces carrot juice
- 4 ounces celery juice
- 2 ounces parsley juice
- 3 ounces spinach juice

Digestive Upset:

- Blend a 2-inch piece of fresh aloe leaf in 16 ounces of pure water

Summer Cooler (in blender):

- Chunks of watermelon or cantaloupe (seeds included)
- Fresh mint (as desired)

Juice for Arthritis:

- 16 ounce of grapefruit juice OR
- 16 ounces of fresh celery juice

Celery Juice:

- Manages diabetic symptoms
- Promotes cardiovascular health
- Relieves migraines and asthma

- Prevents cancer and improves immunity
- Reduces blood pressure and cholesterol
- Prevents urinary tract infections
- Reduces joint pain and swelling

DETOXIFICATION

Detoxification is the process by which your body gets rid of toxins. When you vastly improve your nutrition as happens with juicing, you may experience some symptoms of detox. Detoxification can be unpleasant, so I wanted to talk a bit about the process to equip you in advance should you experience symptoms of detox.

It is ideal to eliminate toxins from your body. When the tissues of your body, typically your fat cells, store toxins, they will eventually wreak havoc. Your body is constantly working on detoxifying itself. As I mentioned above, no matter how clean your lifestyle, you cannot escape toxins. You can minimize your exposure by following my recommendations in this book, but you will always have toxins you have no control over.

We live in a world laden with chemicals—for every American, about thirty thousand pounds of chemicals are produced ever year.[79] You can now ask your doctor to screen you for the chemicals you have in your system. Certain chemicals are more harmful to human health than others, but no chemical lives in your body rent free. For example, a 2007 analysis from the Centers for Disease Control found that 99.7% of American's blood contains C8, otherwise known as perfluorooctanoic acid, or PFOA. This man-made compound is in DuPont's Teflon, in some carpets, and has found its way into drinking water. Results from testing by the Environmental Protection Agency in June 2014, found C8 in ninety-four drinking water systems

---

[79]   https://www.healthline.com/health-news/
test-can-detect-exposure-to-700-everyday-chemicals

that serve 6.5 million Americans.[80] A 2009 study, commissioned by the Environmental Working Group, found two hundred chemicals in minority newborn umbilical cord blood.[81] It can be scary when you realize how toxic our world has become. The point I'm making here is that it is impossible to avoid many toxins in our environment, so we must do what we can to help our body eliminate these toxins. At the same time, we must encourage our elected officials to protect us from such toxins by adopting clean water, air, and food regulations.

Detoxification rarely feels good. Toxins typically feel better going in than they do coming out. Some symptoms of detox include fatigue, skin breakouts, bad breath, foul body odor, nasal discharge, diarrhea, nausea, and more. The organs used to eliminate toxins in your body are the lungs, kidneys, eyes, liver, colon, and tongue. If you feel you are detoxing too fast, you can slow down or halt the process by consuming junk food (which is a toxin, of course). Juice fasting can cause you to dump massive toxins, so some people rarely feel great on a juice fast initially. It really depends on your lifestyle prior to the fast. Stick with it, despite feelings of detox, as you will start to feel amazing soon.

It is important to support your body through the detoxification process by following the advice under the "Instructions for an Efficient Juice Fast" section above. Staying hydrated with lots of pure water, taking rests and naps, incorporating mild exercise such as walking, and making sure your bowels move daily, will all help in the detox process. You can also use techniques such as dry skin brushing, oil pulling, and jumping on a mini trampoline to help the detoxification process. In case you aren't aware of dry skin brushing, it is a technique where

---

[80] https://www.ewg.org/news-insights/news-release/
tiny-concentrations-teflon-chemical-harmful-public-health

[81] https://www.scientificamerican.com/article/
newborn-babies-chemicals-exposure-bpa/

you take a natural stiff-bristled bath brush and massage your skin top to bottom (if you have sensitive skin, you can use a dry washcloth). It helps improve circulation, lymph drainage, and detoxification. You can find resources on the Internet as to the specifics of when and how to dry skin brush. Oil pulling is an ancient Ayurvedic technique that helps fight bacteria in the mouth and can help whiten teeth. It can also pull toxins from the mouth. Simply put one tablespoon of organic coconut oil in your mouth and swish for 20 minutes. Make sure and spit the oil out since you don't want to re-ingest the toxins. Start with 5 minutes a day and work your way up. Stick with the detoxification process because I promise that you will feel better without all the toxins in your body. Your risk for disease will go down, which of course is of paramount importance.

RAW FOOD FASTING

There are other fasts that you can incorporate to improve your health and restore your body to homeostasis. One of my favorite easy fasts to do is a raw food fast. This is a fast where you only consume uncooked food. With both a raw food fast and a juice fast, I recommend doing them in the warmer summer months. You will find it easier to avoid warm food when it's warm outside. This is also a time when you will find an abundance of fresh produce at your local farmer's market.

A raw food fast incorporates raw fruits, vegetables, nuts, and seeds into your diet. You can start the day with a delicious fruit smoothie. For lunch, enjoy a big salad with some sunflower or pumpkin seeds. For dinner, eat another large salad combined with my almond herb dip (in the recipe section) over some spiralized zucchini for a delicious "pasta" type dish. You can also top the noodles with a homemade raw marinara sauce. If you have a powerful blender such as a Vitamix, you can make raw soups.

Eating only raw food for a time will give your digestive system a rest, as it is easier to digest raw food than it is to digest cooked food. Raw food, as we mentioned earlier, is full of enzymes and phytochemicals. A raw food fast is an excellent way to fast without feeling like you are being "cheated." You can even get some raw food crackers made from flaxseeds to help you feel you are eating bread or a cracker. There are excellent raw food restaurants where you can get raw pizza and many other delicious raw food recipes. A great resource with recipes and more is www.fullyraw.com. There is even a Fully Raw app you can download on your phone with wonderful recipes and resources.

INTERMITTENT FASTING

Intermittent fasting has become quite a popular thing lately. It is an eating program that cycles between periods of eating and fasting. There are several intermittent fasts that people use including:

- **The 5/2 diet**—this program allows you to eat normally for five days of the week and on the other two days of your choosing, you only eat 500-600 calories. The two days that you limit calories should not be consecutive days.

- **The 16/8 method**—this method allows you to eat during an eight-hour period during the day and fast the remaining sixteen hours. Many people skip breakfast and eat from 12-8 PM or 1-9 PM.

- **The Eat-Stop-Eat plan**—this method involves going twenty-four hours without eating once or twice a week. People tend to go from dinner one night until dinner the next night.

Intermittent fasting has shown some real benefits, including weight loss. I got introduced to it from my friend Dana, who had struggled with weight issues for years. She lost twenty-five pounds in nine months doing the 5/2 diet consistently.

There are tremendous benefits to allowing your digestive system to rest. As I mentioned earlier, your digestive system is an energy hound. It takes an incredible amount of energy to digest food and assimilate it in the body. Taking time off from eating can free up energy to allow your body to heal. Intermittent fasting allows you the benefits of fasting in an easy-to-do-and-follow plan. Try it, you may like it, especially if you want or need to lose weight.

WATER FASTING

Many experts have used water fasting for extended periods for many reasons. It is one of the most powerful ways to free up energy for your body to cleanse and heal. Clinics like the True North Health Center in Santa Rosa, California, have used water fasting for years to help people regain their health. You can learn more about their programs at www.HealthPromoting.com.

Water fasting can be powerful, but if you water fast for more than a couple of consecutive days, do it under the supervision of a doctor. However, doing a water fast one to two days per week can help kick-start your health in amazing ways. It doesn't matter what day, or days, of the week you choose for water fasting, and they do not have to be the same day each week. Just choose whatever days work best for your schedule. I have found it easier to fast on days I'm busy because the busyness takes my mind off my hungry belly. For several years I water fasted one day per week for spiritual reasons. It was not only a great thing to do spiritually, but it had wonderful physical benefits. I'm just getting back to consistent fasting. It takes discipline but is so worth the effort.

FASTING MIMICKING DIET

The ProLon® Fasting Mimicking Diet® gives many benefits of a water fast while providing delicious food to help fight hunger and protect lean body mass. The company claims you can get a trimmer waistline and many of the associated benefits of fasting without requiring ongoing lifestyle changes, such as long-term dieting (which I never recommend). You purchase their prepackaged foods for the five-day fast. They base the program on twenty years of research sponsored by the National Institutes of Health and conducted at the Longevity Institute and Diabetes and Obesity Research Institute of the University of Southern California (USC). All the foods are plant-based and delicious. The program comes with each day's food and supplements in a box, so it is easy to follow and implement. My husband and I did the program once. I lost four pounds in the five days, and he lost eight pounds. We felt good during the fast, but I did struggle with hunger. Many people have experienced benefits from this program and find it easy to do. You can check it out at www.prolonfast.com.

OTHER FASTS

There are other types of fasts you can do that will benefit you including fasting sugar, processed foods, junk food, alcohol, news, social media, or anything else that seems to control you while not benefiting you. Once you give up something like sugar, I've found you lose your taste buds for it and find it no longer has an appeal. I told my kids when they were growing up and did not like a food, "Don't worry, you get new taste buds every twenty-one days so keep eating it and in three weeks you might like it." [82]

Eating real food is what will help you die young late in life. Just because a product appears in a health food store does not

---

[82]   https://www.alive.com/health/21-days-to-crack-the-code/

mean that it is health-promoting. We have a plethora of processed, organic junk food at our disposal. Once you fast from them, you will find you no longer have the desire to eat them. You can now replace those empty calories with foods that will sustain life and make you feel good.

One of fasting's significant benefits is that it helps to reset your taste buds and helps you to discipline yourself better than almost anything else. If you don't discipline your habits now, your habits will discipline you later. Trust me on that one. The earlier and more often we have discipline over our food choices, the healthier we will be. Step by simple step, you discover that eating a life-giving diet becomes second nature. You reach for an apple instead of a candy bar, or celery instead of chips. I promise you that after a water or juice fast, you will crave healthy plant foods. They will taste like the best chocolate cake you have ever tried. Your body is designed to eat real food. It is the best fuel for your body. Fasting restores your innate desire for healthy, life-giving foods. Incorporate fasting into your life consistently and experience the benefits it gives. You will soon realize that nothing tastes as good as fit and healthy feels! Fasting is worth the effort!

ACTION PLAN

1. **Make a list**—write a list of the things you feel are affecting you negatively, whether it be sugar, alcohol, edible food-like substances, overeating, or social media.

2. **Try a fast**—for just one day a week, fast one of the items on your list. Feel free to go longer than one day but do it for at least a day.

3. **Celebrate progress, not perfection**—for every step you take in a positive direction, give yourself a pat on the back or an "Atta girl or boy." This journey is all about progress and not perfection. As you make changes, you

will get better at sticking with them the longer you go. If you try fasting and make it only an hour, then celebrate it. Try it again another day. No matter what, do not beat yourself up. Be gentle with yourself and celebrate every small win (just do not celebrate with food!).

4. If you have a juicer, make juice at least one day per week. If you don't have a juicer, visit a juice bar in your area and explore various juice combinations. If you are chronically sick, buy a juicer and start juicing daily. It can save your life!

There are several different practices that can help you live all the years you are alive. Routine fasting of various kinds is one of those practices that benefits your body and spirit. We live in a culture of excess that has contributed to an obesity crisis like we've never seen in our history. Taking times to abstain from certain things such as food, junk food, cooked food, television, social media, alcohol, sugar, and the likes will help your physical and spiritual health. One of the best things I recommend is juicing fresh fruits and vegetables. Daily juicing is work but gives your body incredible nutrients that are bioavailable to your cells quickly. I recommend replacing one meal per day with a fresh juice. Juice fasting for one day per week, or three days per quarter, or extended periods, is an incredible gift you can give yourself. It accomplishes the two things necessary to heal your body—nutrients in and toxins out. Start incorporating juicing and fasting in your lifestyle and experience the incredible healing benefits!

STORY TIME: JOHN BEEHNER, FOUNDER OF WISE COUNCIL

(HTTPS://WWW.ASKWISECOUNSEL.COM)

Dr. Deb Harrell "walks her talk." I respect that in any expert and learn more from her each time I am around her. This book is excitingly practical. The body can heal itself. Genesis 1:29 says that "Fruits and vegetables will be our meat." I just turned 80 and feel like I am getting younger following Deb's example and roadmap.

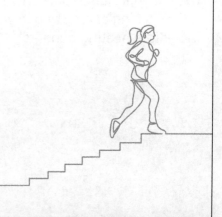

CHAPTER 4

TOXINS OUT

"Plant-based diets are the nutritional
equivalent of quitting smoking."

Neal Barnard, MD

OK, SO HERE comes the chapter you may have been dreading. However, it is a necessary part of our time together. Achieving longevity and quality of life involves what you need to add in (which is by far the most important part), but it is also about what is beneficial for you to take out.

Are you old enough to remember the ads with doctors promoting a particular cigarette brand?[83] There was never any mention that cigarettes harm your health. The implication was that if smoking was good for your doctor, it must be good for you. The ads literally insinuate health benefits from smoking.

It's hard to fathom that anyone would think smoking cigarettes was good for your health in our world today. The

---

[83]   *When Cigarette Companies Used Doctors to Push Smoking,* https://www.history.com/news/cigarette-ads-doctors-smoking-endorsement

evidence is overwhelming to the contrary. The CDC claims on their website that tobacco use is the most preventable cause of disease.[84] But, we all know that, even smokers. They put a very large label on all cigarette packs stating the warning that cigarettes harm your health. Unfortunately, many people still spend big bucks to suck in something that most likely will give them cancer. Tobacco is extremely addictive. If you smoke, please consider doing whatever is necessary to give up the habit. It may eventually kill you and will diminish your quality of life, not to mention make you age very rapidly. I can always tell a smoker by their skin.

Why am I talking about smoking here? The point I'm making is that just because the experts, aka medical professionals, don't tell you to stop eating the things I'm going to be talking about next, does not mean they are a healthy food for you. You can't always trust the "experts" as the smoking situation demonstrated. How many lives could have been saved had cigarettes not come with the endorsement of doctors? I imagine quite a lot. Please reread Dr. Neal Barnard's quote above just under the chapter heading.

DITCH THE DAIRY

I bet you remember the "Milk—It Does a Body Good" ad campaign with celebrities sporting milk mustaches. Then there was the "Got Milk?" campaign, again with celebrities sporting white mustaches. The claims these ads make are false. They claimed things like— dairy builds strong bones, helps you lose weight, is necessary for kids to grow big and strong, etc. If you look at the preponderance of scientific research, you find that cow's milk turns cancer on in the body, provides a negative calcium balance to the body (which causes osteoporosis—the countries that consume the most dairy products

---

[84] Smoking: The Most Preventable Cause of Disease, https://www.cdc.gov/museum/online/story-of-cdc/smoking/

have significantly higher rates of osteoporosis), is acidic to the body, is a mucous producer, and can cause acne, to name a few things.[8586] "Milk—It Does a Body Bad" is what the slogan would tout if it was speaking the truth.

Dr. T. Colin Campbell, PhD researcher from Cornell University, discovered in his fifty years of extensive nutritional research looking at nutrition and cancer, that the protein in dairy turns cancer on in the body. For details about his research and results, I highly recommend you read his books, *The China Study* and *Whole*. Also check out the documentary titled "Forks Over Knives." You can watch it for free at https://www.forksoverknives.com/the-film/.

Do you realize we are the only species that drinks another species milk? We are also the only species that continues drinking milk after the weaning age. Milk is the ideal food for a baby calf—it is "baby calf growth fluid," as Michael Klaper, MD, calls it.[87] It is not for humans! Think about it, every time you drink milk or eat yogurt or cheese, you are taking milk from a baby calf. Not to mention the milk industry is riddled with torture and sadness. Please realize that in order to keep that female cow lactating (so humans can take her milk), some horrific stuff happens.

Within a day after the calf is born, it is removed from the mother causing tremendous grief on both the calf and its mom. As a mom who nursed my babies, I can't imagine the horror of that. Where do the babies go? Males typically are either sent to barren, filthy feedlots awaiting slaughter or

---

85   https://www.pcrm.org/news/news-releases/fda-sued-ignoring-petition-calling-breast-cancer-warning-labels-cheese

86   *12 Frightening Facts About Milk*, https://nutritionstudies.org/12-frightening-facts-milk/

87   Michael Klaper, MD, https://www.youtube.com/watch?v=Wpc8yH_V-AI

used for veal after about two months of being held in a cage that keeps them from standing. Companies do this to keep them from developing muscles, so the veal is "tender." The baby females usually become dairy cows, sadly. Poor calves, alone and frightened and robbed of their moms.

To get the lactating cow to continue producing milk under these horrific circumstances, they often pump her full of hormones. The average cow today produces up to four times the amount of milk than cows did in 1950. This over-production does not happen naturally. It is because they are being given growth hormones, so they produce more milk for people, not their young. And since they hook her up to a milking machine several times per day, she often develops mastitis and is fed antibiotics. These antibiotics, hormones, and pus from her teats pass through in the milk to unaware consumers.[88] Feel free to look up how much pus is allowed in milk from the link provided in the footnote if you find this hard to believe.[89]

Cows typically live about twenty years when conditions are normal. They kill dairy cows after about four to five years because their bodies wear out from constantly being pregnant or lactating. Did you know that a cow is pregnant for nine months, just like humans? Exhausted dairy cows are turned into soup for humans, dog and cat food, or ground beef. Nearly fifty percent of dairy cows are lame by the time of their execution from standing on concrete floors and intensive confinement, as reported in a dairy industry study.[90]

Do you in good conscience believe that the Creator of the universe really wants His creatures treated this way? The

---

88   https://headlines.peta.org/take-action-help-cows-dairy-industry/

89   Michael Greger, MD, *How Much Pus is There in Milk?*, https://nutrition-facts.org/2011/09/08/how-much-pus-is-there-in-milk/

90   https://www.peta.org/issues/animals-used-for-food/factory-farming/cows/dairy-industry/

Bible clearly states in Proverbs 12:10 MSG, "Good people are good to their animals; the 'good-hearted' bad people kick and abuse them." I can promise you that the way dairy gets to your table involves more abuse than you care to consider, or I bet would agree to. I constantly wonder why God does not intervene (oh yeah, He gave us free will—more on that later) and put a stop to this and other insanity in our world. This horrific torturous industry exists because of one thing— greed! The Merriam Webster dictionary defines greed as, "a selfish and excessive desire for more of something than is needed."[91] This greed comes from the industries producing these products, and greed by the people consuming them. The industry desires more profits at whatever cost and the consumers desire more dairy products at whatever savings. Please do not stick your head in the sand and pretend that ignorance is bliss. It is not. This hormone and antibiotic filled milk, cheese, yogurt and whey protein is wreaking havoc on your body even if you don't realize it right now. I'm sorry to be so blunt, but I am committed to be the bearer of truth and help you and these animals avoid suffering.

I encourage you to educate yourself on dairy products and how they arrive in your belly. Both www.PETA.org and www. farmsanctuary.org have good info on the industry. I warn you; the photos and videos are disturbing. I beg you to not turn a blind eye to the abuse of God's creatures. My burden to see this suffering end is enormous and is one of the major reasons I do what I do. I encourage you to ditch the dairy and notice the difference. It has never been easier to eliminate dairy with all the great options for plant-based milks, cheese, and yogurt. It will amaze you. One of my young clients gave up dairy recently and noticed her chronic digestive issues and acne cleared up. I have seen many people experience an improvement in their health from ditching dairy. From my

---

[91]   https://www.merriam-webster.com/dictionary/greed

own experience, once you go without dairy for a couple of months, you will not like the taste of it anymore.

However, be aware that dairy is addicting as you break the habit. It has casomorphins (casein-derived morphine-like compounds) in it that can attach to the same brain receptors that heroin and other narcotics attach to. These opiates are in milk to reward the baby for nursing. They are also in human breast milk, which is why a baby is often calm after nursing. To learn more about casomorphins and dairy, I highly recommend reading Dr. Neal Barnard's book, *The Cheese Trap.*[92]

Here are a few of my non-dairy favorites to help you break the animal dairy habit:

- Cashew milk (to make your own, blend 1/8 cup raw cashews and 8 ounces of water in a high-powered blender), oat, almond or soy milk

- Follow Your Heart, Violife, and Chao sliced cheeses

- Miyoko's soft "cheeses"

- Trader Joe's vegan coconut milk ice cream—yummy! Other brands are good too. However, these should only be used for a special occasion as they are still junk food!

- Violife shreds for pizza, etc. This brand melts the best. Or simply make my cashew "cheeze" recipe in Chapter 7

- Daiya Greek style yogurt. Violife cream cheese is yummy, and I bet you will not be able to tell it from cow's milk cream cheese.

---

[92] Neal Barnard, MD, *The Cheese Trap–How Breaking a Surprising Addiction Will Help You Lose Weight, Gain Energy, and Get Healthy,* (Hachette Book Group, 2017)

- Follow Your Heart or Forager sour cream or make your own by blending 1/2 cup of raw cashews + 3/4 cup of water + 2 tablespoons of lemon juice + 1/2 teaspoon of miso. Allow to sit on the counter for up to 36 hours. This will culture the mixture and it will have a sour cream taste and feel.

Interesting Facts About Cows:

- They have a memory of three years
- They have best friends
- Love to play

Compliments of the Humane League

CHOOSE COMPASSIONATE HEART-HEALTHY PROTEIN

Meat. Another obsession, especially with the incredible marketing of the Paleo and Ketogenic camps. These groups promote their diets with vengeance and lack of scientific evidence. Much "science" that is out there is junk science. Again, follow the money. The very industry of the products tested fund a lot of the research. For example, you can learn about the "benefits" of dairy from the dairy council, the "benefits" of eggs from the egg council, etc. Look at who funds the research and who benefits from its results.

Biblically, you may eat animals. Eating them is not a spiritual issue. It is a physical issue, and the last time I checked, you need your body to get around on this planet. Yes, your spirit lives on past this earth, but should you be as healthy as you can, and live as long as possible so that you can positively affect your world? This requires good stewardship of your body. Science conclusively shows a link between meat consumption and disease.[93]

Even eating the animals that God clearly said not to eat in the Levitical dietary laws—such as pigs, shellfish, insects, and birds of prey—is allowed, spiritually that is. Physically, it's not a good idea. I tell people, "Eating bacon will not keep you out of Heaven. In fact, it will get you there that much quicker." Smile, unless you love bacon and ham and sausage and hot dogs and all things pig. You might not smile if that is the case. Eating bacon in everything from chocolate chip cookies to chips to bourbon has become the fad. You can thank the National Pork Producers Council for that. They represent the approximately sixty thousand pork producers in America by influencing legislation, marketing their wares, and persuading people to buy their products. They work diligently to overcome the challenges brought about by organizations like the World Health Organization, who warned in 2015 that processed meats like bacon, sausage and hot dogs are carcinogenic—they cause cancer.[94] They also stated that meats like beef, pork, lamb, and veal are "probably carcinogenic too." WHO put eating processed meats in the same category of smoking cigarettes and being exposed to asbestos. Gulp! You can imagine the hit that must have taken on pork producers and why the council "beefed" up its efforts to market its products to consumers in everything from cookies to bourbon.

This book is not about debating Scripture with you, it's about helping you reclaim your health based on solid science and results I have witnessed. What do we know about animal food consumption? Let's look to the blue zones for guidance,

---

[93] https://www.ox.ac.uk/news/2021-03-02-regular-meat-consumption-linked-wide-range-common-diseases

[94] https://www.hsph.harvard.edu/nutritionsource/2015/11/03/report-says-eating-processed-meat-is-carcinogenic-understanding-the-findings/

those areas where people normally live to be over one hundred in disability-free health. Dan Buettner, the author of *Blue Zones-9 Lessons for Living Longer from the People Who've Lived the Longest,* boiled down the habits that all these zones had in common. They were all predominantly plant-based, meaning ninety to one hundred percent of calories come from plant foods. Animal products were kept to a minimum, if eaten at all.[95]

We also know that a plant-based diet is the only diet proven not only to prevent cardiovascular disease, but to reverse it. Thanks to the works of Dr. Caldwell Esselstyn and Dr. Dean Ornish, many people have reversed this disease using a low-fat vegan diet.[96] Countless have avoided open heart surgery and stints (both of which have nasty side effects and are quite radical), and toxic medicines that do little to improve the situation. Thanks to the work of these and other doctors such as Joel Kahn, MD, and Jamie Dulaney, MD, willing participants are healing their hearts through plant-based nutrition. My thought is that if a plant-based diet helps you live longer and better, and reverses advanced heart disease (again the number one killer of both men and women), why not follow it for prevention?

It turns out that avoiding animals as food helps a host of other conditions as well: type-one diabetes, cancer, arthritis, auto-immune disorders, digestive issues, lung disease, kidney disease, brain disorders such as Alzheimer's, and Parkinson's

---

[95] Dan Buettner, *The Blue Zones-9 Lessons for Living Longer From the People Who've Lived the Longest,* (National Geographic, 2012)

[96] Dean Ornish, MD, *Dr. Dean Ornish's Program For Reversing Heart Disease: The Only System Scientifically Proven to Reverse Heart Disease Without Drugs or Surgery,* (Ivy Books, 1995) & Caldwell Esselstyn, MD, *Prevent and Reverse Heart Disease: The Revolutionary, Scientifically Proven, Nutrition-Based Cure,* (Avery Publisher, 2008)

disease.[97] There are many books by reputable doctors using plant-based diets to heal people. You can find all the scientific information you want in those books. I include my complete list of suggested resources and books in Chapter 6 titled Thrival Guide.

Isabel is a one of my best friends. She is a beautiful and loving Cuban American with a sweet husband and four kids. She is a busy real estate agent and an excellent cook. She called me a couple of years ago to ask my advice when she had dangerously high blood pressure, to the point of being hospitalized. She committed to make dietary changes to improve her health and get off of the four blood pressure pills each day for her excessively high blood pressure. I persuaded her to switch to a whole-foods plant-based diet with little to no oil. She switched immediately and within six months on a healthy vegan diet, she was down to much less medicine. She began making time for exercise and rest, and as they say, the rest is history. See below her story in her words.

Let's talk about how animals get to your plate so you can know what the process involves. It is difficult for me to write about this because it grieves me so, but I feel for you to make your best decision, you need all the facts.

Let's start with chicken, or the "holy" bird, as my husband calls it. They kill approximately nine billion (9,000,000,000) chickens for their meat each year and about 300,000,000 (that's 300 million) are used for egg production. Chickens are being bred for hyper-production, which involves messing with their genes and manipulating their bodies with hormones. Chickens are the most numerous of animals raised for food and are some of the most abused.[98]

---

[97] https://www.ncbi.nlm.nih.gov/pmc/articles/PMC3662288/

[98] https://www.peta.org/issues/animals-used-for-food/factory-farming/chickens/

The average meat chicken (and turkey) lives indoors in large sheds. Companies cram twenty thousand or more on a single level, causing them to have to live in their waste, which causes high ammonia concentration that burns their eyes, throats, and skin. They keep the lights on for almost twenty-four hours to keep chickens eating and growing. To make matters worse, when a chicken dies (and many do because of the stress), they leave the dead chicken in with the live ones, causing even more stress and hygiene issues.

We had two hens a few years ago for pets. They are very social and make great pets, and the ticks and fleas in our yard were non-existent with them foraging. We also never had fire ants during those years. Bonus! It took about four months before they reached full maturity and started laying eggs (my dogs were happy to enjoy their eggs). However, in factory farms, because of breeding and growth hormones, chickens reach maturity in six weeks versus four months. In 1925, it took sixteen weeks to raise a chicken to 2.5 pounds. Today chickens weigh double that in six weeks. Because of these practices, chickens grow disproportionately and quickly, with larger breasts in order to meet market demand. This often leads to weak legs, breathing problems, and heart failure. Many cannot support their bodies with their legs and as a result cannot reach food and water.[99]

Egg-laying hens don't have it any better, in fact they may have it worse. They spend their lives in a similar shed to chickens used for meat but in battery cages that are the size of a file drawer. They keep up to ten hens in each cage. These cages provide floor space in the amount of less than an 8.5-inch by 11-inch sheet of paper. Think about that. They are so stressed by the lack of space that they become aggressive and attack their fellow cage-mates. The breeders remedy that situation by burning or slicing off a piece of their beaks (with

---

[99]   https://thehumaneleague.org/article/factory-farmed-chickens

no painkillers). When the hen's egg production slows because of age, breeders often withhold nourishment for up to two weeks to force a final laying. After that, the hen is no longer needed. They will kill some right on the farm. Others will go to slaughter where their battered bodies become food scraps. I won't talk about the slaughter process.

Many consumers are choosing brands that have "free-range" written on them, and that's great, however, you cannot trust that label.[100] The only label you can really trust is the "Animal Welfare Approved" label.[101] If you decide after reading this book you want to continue eating eggs, I suggest finding a farmer you know and visit their farm to verify the humane treatment of the birds.

Interesting Facts About Chickens:

- Have different vocalizations for different objects
- See more colors than people can
- Can count to ten
- Can plan for the future
- Can differentiate human faces

Compliments of the Humane League

I'm sure you have seen the bumper sticker, "Beef—it's what's for dinner." Or the one that says, "Real men eat beef." Perhaps you've seen the one that I find most offensive, "Beef—what vegetarians eat when they cheat." These marketing slogans came about because of the sharp decline in beef consumption thanks to organizations like the World Health Organization saying that it probably causes cancer—see above.

---

[100]   https://thegrownetwork.com/raising-chickens-factory-farms/

[101]   https://agreenerworld.org/certifications/animal-welfare-approved/

Unfortunately, close to thirty million cows are killed annually in the United States for food. They brand and castrate cows and may have their horns removed, all without painkillers.[102] If you are a man, imagine being castrated without anesthesia. Or being castrated at all! Right! Cows typically spend a lot of their lives outdoors. For the last several months of their lives however, most cows live in feedlots where they are crammed with hundreds of thousands of other cows until they are slaughtered. These feedlots do not provide pasture or shelter, and therefore the cows must stand in their own waste and are subject to harsh elements. I have passed by feedlots in Texas and Oklahoma—the stench is overwhelming and an incredibly sad site to see. I have heard people in those areas say of the smell, "Smells like money to me." How very sad to have that disregard for the lives of sentient beings. Cows are gentle creatures that have a social network like that of dogs.

Lastly, I want to tell you about pigs. I mentioned earlier how unhealthy they are to eat. In case the temptation to eat ham and bacon is still with you, let me tell you about their sad lives. They perhaps have the worst fate of the factory farmed animals, believe it or not. It's hard to imagine anything worse than what I've already talked about. But it gets worse, sadly!

Pigs are very smart animals. They are more intelligent than dogs, and researchers have ranked them above three-year-old children as far as intelligence.[103] The United States raises about one hundred million pigs each year for food, and they raise the majority on factory farms. Over ninety-seven percent of pigs spend their lives indoors with no room to move. Because they cannot do what pigs do naturally—root

---

[102] https://www.peta.org/issues/animals-used-for-food/factory-farming/cows/

[103] https://www.peta.org/issues/animals-used-for-food/animals-used-food-factsheets/pigs-intelligent-animals-suffering-factory-farms-slaughterhouses/

around in the earth, etc.—they become depressed and anxious and will bite the other pigs crammed in the small indoor space with them. They often bite the other pig's tails off, therefore the farmers cut their tails off (with no anesthesia) to avoid this happening. They also break baby pig's teeth in half, remove male pig's testicles, and perform ear notching, again with no anesthesia.[104]

Unfortunately, pigs raised on "free-range" and "humane" farms often still get castrated, and their ears notched, with no anesthesia. They also often have nose rings put in their noses to keep them from rooting around in the dirt because the farmers say it ruins the pasture. Experts consider rooting an essential welfare need of every pig. The rings make it uncomfortable for them to root, which frustrates them. They are trying to keep these animals from acting the way God created them to act. All so people can enjoy eating their flesh.

Would you consider eating your dog or cat? If not, why? Why eat cows and not dogs and cats? (They eat dogs in some countries, sadly.) Why eat chickens and not dogs and cats? I mean, an animal is an animal. Not that I am advocating eating dogs and cats. I'm advocating not eating any animals, or very little if you feel you must have some meat. There is no reason to consume animals when there are so many nutritious plant-based options at your disposal. It is a horrible use of resources, is detrimental to the environment, and involves untold torture.

If this all sounds unacceptable to you, consider tacit agreement. Every single time you buy one of these animal products, you tacitly agree with the practices that got that animal to your plate. You vote with your wallet. The only way these inhumane treatments will ever stop is if people stop

---

[104] https://www.peta.org/issues/animals-used-for-food/factory-farming/pigs/

purchasing the products. Vote with your wallet and please stop this insanity.

I believe it is our responsibility as citizens of this planet to make sure we do not contribute to this horror. Please, for the sake of your health, our planet, and these poor creatures, avoid animals as food. Choose healthier, compassionate, plant-based options. You will be glad you did; I promise. This book will help you make the switch.

STORY TIME: ISABEL RODRIGUEZ

"Deb has been instrumental the last twenty years of my life helping me establish a healthy diet and lifestyle. When I say diet, I'm not referring to a diet geared to losing weight, although that will naturally happen, but a lifestyle choosing the right foods to nourish your body. Several years ago, I was faced with the fear of taking up to four prescription medications for high blood pressure, which was not the road I wanted to take. So, after talking late that evening with Deb, I went "COLD" turkey to a vegan lifestyle. I had eaten mostly vegetarian for several years before but cutting dairy and the occasional organic meat still made a huge difference. I now take only one small dosage and one-half of another small dosage of medication. The only reason I do that is I'm a realtor and my personality and business do interact, and I haven't figured out yet how to be calm at times in a high stress career! I plan to fully go without medicine in the next few years when I retire. As a businesswoman, I thought it was going to be too difficult to become vegan but through Deb's help and research I've found it very easy to do. Deb has shared numerous recipes and has always been a listening ear full of wisdom and information, not only for me but issues dealing with my children along the way as well. One of the many attributes that I love about Deb is that she doesn't judge you; she provides facts, lots of love, as well as support. If you are looking for a life coach and friend to help you navigate the whole-food plant-based approach, there could be no better advocate than Dr. Deb Harrell."

JUST SAY NO TO SUGAR

We can categorize refined sugar as a poison (Webster's Dictionary describes a poison as "something destructive or harmful"[105]), and an addictive drug rather than food, as it does not provide any nutrition to the body and robs nutrients from the body, especially from the teeth and bones. Sugar is also harmful to the stomach lining and interferes with digestion. I classify it as an anti-nutrient because it requires more nutrients in the body to process it than it gives the body. Sugar is addictive, causes drastic mood swings, and has withdrawal symptoms like a drug.[106]

In 2019, the average American consumed 72.7 pounds of sugar a year, down from 89.3 pounds per person in 1999. That is the equivalent of approximately seventeen teaspoons per day.[107] Soft drink consumption comprises thirty-three percent of sugar eaten by adults. In one twenty-ounce soda, there are about seventeen teaspoons of sugar. Wow! Virtually all processed foods have sugar in them, including processed fruits and vegetables. Start reading labels and it will surprise you at what contains sugar, and how much! Realize that four grams of sugar equals about one teaspoon.

Sugar provides empty calories. Empty calories give no nutritional benefit to your body. One gram of sugar is equal to four calories, so that twenty-ounce soda (sixty-eight grams) will contain two hundred seventy-two calories from sugar. It's always best to consume nutrient-dense calories—ones that provide an abundance of nutrients per calorie. Besides

---

[105]   https://www.merriam-webster.com/dictionary/poison

[106]   https://www.huffpost.com/entry/dangers-of-sugar_b_3658061

[107]   https://www.sugar.org/diet/intake/

providing calories with zero nutrients, sugar wreaks havoc in the body in the following ways:[108]

- Kills the good bacteria in your gut
- Decreases the efficiency of the immune system
- Causes dental decay
- Contributes to weight gain and obesity
- Weakens bones because of acidity
- Can cause moodiness and emotional imbalance
- Contributes to ADD/ADHD
- Is Inflammatory
- Contributes to blood pressure issues
- Contributes to fatty liver disease

I am not suggesting that you never indulge in an occasional sugary treat. It's not what you do occasionally that will affect your health on a large scale, but what you do regularly. Occasionally having something sweet is fine. Just be careful not to overindulge because sugar is very addicting. (If you know you are a sugar addict, you may want to abstain from *processed* sugar altogether.) Having the occasional piece of birthday cake or cookie should not hurt you. Just reserve sugar for special occasions. I am warning you though that once you give up sugar, you might not like the taste of it.

I suggest you avoid **agave nectar**. This has gained a lot of popularity in the last few years, but it's not a health food as they would have you believe. Agave syrup is likened to nature's high fructose corn syrup. It even has more fructose than high fructose corn syrup. It spikes your insulin and can affect your hormones. It's best to avoid it.

There are healthier options for special treats than refined sugar. The healthiest option is fruit. As I mentioned in the

---

[108] https://www.health.harvard.edu/heart-health/the-sweet-danger-of-sugar

prior chapter, the best way to satisfy your sweet tooth is with fruit. Not only does it contain natural sugars, but fruit also contains lots of nutrients, so it's a nutrient-dense food. Dried fruits like dates, dried apricots, raisins, figs, and the likes are a great sweet treat.

My Suggested Sweeteners:

- **Date sugar**—a great substitute for baking but it can be expensive.

- **Coconut sugar**—When I make a birthday cake for someone or cookies during the holidays, I prefer using coconut sugar (or monk fruit sweetener). Coconut sugar tastes like brown sugar, but contains antioxidants, vitamins, and minerals unlike white sugar. It also has a lower glycemic index than refined sugar, keeping your blood sugar and insulin levels steadier.

- **Monk fruit sweetener**—This is a sweetener that has become popular recently and comes from the lo han guo fruit, which is a small melon that grows in China and Thailand. They often combine it with erythritol (an alcohol sweetener) in products, but you can find it alone, which is the way I prefer it. They have used monk fruit as a sweetener and herbal remedy for centuries in the East. Monk fruit extract is safe for diabetics, has zero calories, and is generally recognized as safe by the FDA. It does not have the aftertaste that stevia has for some people, and you can't tell the difference between monk fruit extract and sugar in baking. It provides 150-200 times the sweetness of sugar without the negatives associated with sugar. Look for pure monk fruit extract.

- **Stevia**—I also like to bake using stevia although some people don't like the taste of stevia in baked goods. The brand of stevia I use is Enzo Organic Stevia. They have a conversion table on the back of their bag of stevia. One cup of sugar is equal to four teaspoons of Enzo stevia. Enzo has a more concentrated version of stevia (3125 servings per bag) that I use for sweetening my tea, but the less concentrated one is great for baking (1600 servings per bag).

MINIMIZE ALCOHOL

I know, here I go again. At this point you may not consider me your friend, but trust me, I am! It is important to understand the pros and cons of alcohol so you can make informed decisions about whether to consume it. There are plenty of studies showing that moderate alcohol consumption can have some benefits, especially for the heart. For example, if you look at the data from the blue zones, one to two small glasses of red wine per day is often a part of most of these communities that have the longest-lived people in the world.[109] We don't know if the alcohol consumption provides some protection or if the benefit is more attributed to the fact that they drink that alcohol with other people, and the community aspect provides the benefit.

Other studies show that daily alcohol consumption, even one drink per day, can cause cancer. Here's what Dr. Greger says regarding alcohol and cancer on his video dated March 28, 2018, titled "Can Alcohol Cause Cancer?":

"We've known about the possible association between the consumption of alcohol and excessive mortality from cancer for more than a hundred years. Though the evidence is accumulating that alcohol drinking is also associated with pancreatic cancer, prostate cancer, and melanoma, we're pretty certain that alcohol increases risk of mouth cancer, throat cancer,

---

[109] *Longevity Link: How Wine Helps You Live Longer,* https://www.bluezones.com/2017/08/longevity-link-how-and-why-wine-helps-you-live-longer/

esophageal cancer, colorectal cancer, liver cancer, voice-box cancer, and breast cancer. Current estimates suggest that alcohol causes about 5.8% of all cancer deaths in these organs worldwide. Here's how that breaks down for men and women. In men, alcohol causes mostly head and neck cancers, and gastrointestinal cancers, whereas it's mostly breast cancer in women. Alcohol appears to cause more than 100,000 cases of breast cancer every year. Yeah, but is that just among heavy drinkers? No. All levels of evidence show...a risk relationship between alcohol consumption and the risk of breast cancer, even at low levels of consumption. Now, eating a healthy diet may help modulate that risk. Yeah, alcohol increases the risk of breast cancer, but 'a fiber-rich diet [may have] the opposite effect.' So, eating more whole plant foods may be able to 'ease the adverse effects' of alcohol. Alcohol has been shown to increase sex hormone levels, like estrogen, which may increase breast cancer risk. But you see the opposite happen eating fiber-rich foods. Fiber [appears to] bind estrogen in the colon and help flush it out of the body. **But, even so, there does not appear to be any level of alcohol consumption that is completely safe from a cancer standpoint.**"[110]

Here's what The National Cancer Institute (www.cancer.gov) says: "Researchers have hypothesized multiple ways that alcohol may increase the risk of cancer, including:

- metabolizing (breaking down) ethanol in alcoholic drinks to acetaldehyde, which is a toxic chemical and a probable human carcinogen; acetaldehyde can damage both DNA (the genetic material that makes up genes) and proteins

- generating reactive oxygen species (chemically reactive molecules that contain oxygen), which can damage

---

[110] https://nutritionfacts.org/video/can-alcohol-cause-cancer/

DNA, proteins, and lipids (fats) in the body through a process called oxidation

- impairing the body's ability to break down and absorb a variety of nutrients that may be associated with cancer risk, including vitamin A; nutrients in the vitamin B complex, such as folate; vitamin C; vitamin D; vitamin E; and carotenoids

- increasing blood levels of <u>estrogen</u>, a sex hormone linked to the risk of breast cancer

Alcoholic beverages may also contain a variety of carcinogenic contaminants that are introduced during fermentation and production, such as nitrosamines, asbestos fibers, phenols, and hydrocarbons."[111]

Of course, we all know people who drink daily and live to a ripe old age. My mom was an example of that. She lived to ninety drinking every day. Her quality of life in her last several years was less than ideal though. And she developed breast cancer, which did not kill her but made her uncomfortable for the last ten years of her life (she received no treatment for it). There will always be people who "beat the odds" but do you want to gamble on being one of the few who beat the odds?

Consistent alcohol consumption is linked to poor sleep, brain shrinkage from heavy usage, indigestion, stomach ulcers, kidney issues, liver disease, pancreas damage and diabetes, gout, dehydration, an offbeat heart, high blood pressure, weakened immune system, hormonal issues in both men and women, hearing loss, and thinning bones. Are you sure you want that drink now?

---

[111] *Alcohol and Cancer Risk*, <u>https://www.cancer.gov/about-cancer/causes-prevention/risk/alcohol/alcohol-fact-sheet</u>

Alcohol is acidic to the body (hence the thinning of bones), provides mostly empty calories, and can contain pesticides, additives, and other undesirables which are not optimal for your health. For example, most beer and many wines contain glyphosate, the nasty chemical in Roundup and what they spray on genetically modified crops to kill the weeds (but it does not kill the crop because of the genetic modification).[112] They have linked Roundup to Parkinson's disease, cancer, and infertility in studies, yet the United States continues to allow its use, sadly.[113] There are many other synthetic pesticides, fungicides, insecticides, and fertilizers used in the production of grapes for wine, and grains for beer and other alcohol. Unfortunately, many of these contaminants pass through to the final product.

If you choose to consume alcohol, I recommend the following:

1. Choose Non-GMO Verified alcohol to avoid glyphosate, or organic to avoid glyphosate and synthetic pesticides, fungicides, insecticides, and fertilizers.

2. Drink occasionally—only a couple of drinks per week. Remember daily alcohol consumption is linked to higher cancer risk as well as many other undesirables!

3. When drinking, have a glass of water in between every alcoholic drink to keep you from drinking too much and to help you stay hydrated.

4. Eat a healthy snack before or during your cocktails.

The principal thing to remember is that alcohol is not a health food. Use it in moderation, and by moderation, I mean only occasionally. Reserve it for special occasions and limit the

---

[112] https://livelovefruit.com/glyphosate-in-beer-and-wine/

[113] https://beyondpesticides.org/dailynewsblog/2020/05/glyphosate-in-roundup-linked-to-parkinsons-disease/

amount you drink in one setting to avoid hangovers. When I stopped drinking several years ago, I found I was more attached to the idea of drinking than the drinking itself. Although there were times when I was younger that I drank way too much, mostly I had become a moderate drinker with only a couple of glasses of wine when I indulged. The way I felt each time I drank motivated me to stop drinking. Even though I only had a couple of drinks, I would wake up in the middle of the night and feel dizzy. It also really bothered my stomach if I drank for consistent days, like on vacation. I decided my body was telling me to stop. I have felt so much better since eliminating alcohol from my lifestyle. Now if I am with people who are drinking socially, I will often have kombucha in a wine glass or just water. It gives me the same satisfaction of drinking alcohol without the negative side effects.

ACTION PLAN

1. Try PCRM's 21-Day Vegan Kickstart—you can do anything for twenty-one days. They have a free app that you can download on your phone complete with recipes, daily encouragement, shopping lists, etc. Keep a journal of how you feel each day. At the beginning, record all your physical symptoms. At the end, note how your symptoms changed or disappeared over the twenty-one days. Hopefully at the end, it will motivate you to keep going!

2. Minimize your alcohol consumption. If you drink daily, try only indulging on the weekend. Follow the suggestions I mentioned in that section for each time you drink. Note how you feel physically and emotionally. Journal about your relationship with alcohol.

3. Purchase one of my suggested sweeteners and make one of my dessert recipes in chapter 7. Start eating fruit when you crave something sweet instead of grabbing

candy or other sugary items you are used to eating. Journal about your relationship with sugar.

4. Try one of the cheese and dairy alternatives I mentioned. Ditch the dairy for twenty-one days and notice how you feel.

We live in an increasingly toxic world which is undermining our health, and the health of this beautiful planet we call home. Getting the toxins out of your diet is a key component for healing. Science has shown that eating lower on the food chain minimizes the toxic load to the body. There are none of us that would challenge the well-known fact that cigarettes are harmful to human health, now. However, back in the 1950's, people assumed smoking cigarettes was a healthy habit and doctors even promoted specific brands. The preponderance of scientific evidence is now showing that animal products are not health promoting, despite (like cigarettes in the fifties) doctors promoting them. Consuming animal products is taking a toll on human health, on the animals being treated inhumanely, and on the planet. Ingesting excessive alcohol and sugar are also contributing to the toxic load placed on the body. I urge you to choose healthier, compassionate, and more environmentally friendly options, and experience better health and longevity.

CHAPTER 5

WINNING THE INNER GAME AND OTHER COMPONENTS TO HEALTH

"And most of all I will love myself. For when I do, I will zealously inspect all things which enter my body, my mind, my soul, and my heart. Never will I overindulge the requests of my flesh, rather I will cherish my body with cleanliness and moderation. Never will I allow my mind to be attracted to evil and despair, rather I will uplift it with the knowledge and wisdom of the ages. Never will I allow my soul to become complacent and satisfied, rather I will feed it with meditation and prayer. Never will I allow my heart to become small and bitter, rather I will share it and it will grow and warm the earth."

Og Mandino

IT IS IMPERATIVE to incorporate the components in this chapter in order to flourish—body, soul and spirit. Good nutrition alone, although a significant component to health, will most likely not make you one-hundred percent healthy and vibrant, long-term. It's crucial to address your thoughts, exercise your body, stay hydrated, connect with your purpose, and more. I hope you enjoy this chapter. I know aspects of it may challenge some, but I hope you will put in the effort to work through these components of health. Their importance cannot be overstated!

BEGIN WITH THE END IN MIND

I was having a conversation one day with a couple of younger women about my lifestyle. They had commented on how good I looked for my age. I told them I felt it was because of my plant-based and active lifestyle that I have been at for so long (forty-four years as of our conversation). They both commented on how they just could not give up meat or cheese. Many people have the same mindset, and don't even want to consider giving up these foods.

I was contemplating the conversation later, and it came to me that the issue with the mindset most people have regarding health and nutrition, is that they are not beginning with the end in mind. In Stephen Covey's *Seven Habits of Highly Effective People* book, he lists this as one of the seven habits that highly successful people have.[114] In coaching someone the other day who is struggling with adopting healthy habits, I suggested the same thing to her—that she begin with the end in mind. Many people don't think that much about their habits until negative results surface. Then they look at changing their diet, starting to exercise, etc. Beginning with the end in mind can avoid so much suffering.

---

[114] Stephen R. Covey, *The 7 Habits of Highly Effective People*, (Simon & Schuster, 2013)

One of the major reasons I practice self-care is that I am beginning with the end of my life in mind, which I hope will be many years down the road. I want to be active and self-sufficient my entire life. Honestly, I don't want my kids to need to take care of me. Not because I think they would not want to do it, but because I just don't want them to have to. I'd rather be vibrant all the years I'm alive. Realize that your future health starts right now. What do you want it to look like? Do you want to have energy? Do you want to be fit? Do you want to do all the things you want to do for years to come, or be limited because of physical illness? I encourage you to make your health decisions based on the results you envision. Be willing to invest now for a great payoff later, instead of gambling that your choices won't matter. Begin with the end in mind. Helane's story is a testimony to the power of investing in your health!

STORY TIME: HELANE DAVIS

Helane has lived her life with the end in mind.

"As a nonagenarian, I can gratefully reflect on the good Lord's divine appointment. A couple decades ago, Dr. Deb Harrell walked across the parking lot to my car the very next day after I had pleadingly prayed to somehow be connected to her. My heart's yearning was for a doctor, who in addition to having a heart for the Lord, also had a passion for prevention. Repeatedly and very patiently, Deb has encouraged me with practical (i.e., eat the rainbow) guidelines that have consistently been accompanied by impactful educational materials and prayer. Despite my occasional inconsistencies, Deb never ever gave up on me. First, she would firmly help me identify the cause for 'backsliding', and then I could always depend on Deb to graciously, consistently, and straight-forwardly help me re-implement the sound principles of God's basic divine design for getting and maintaining good health. Due to Deb's loving wisdom, I am experiencing a new level of self-nurturing and stewardship over the health God is allowing me as a joyful, very grateful 93-year young woman."

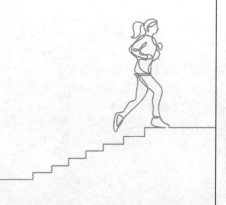

TFAR = THOUGHTS FEELINGS ACTIONS RESULTS

"I was constantly trying to think myself into a new way of living instead of loving myself into a new way of thinking."

Brennan Manning

One way many people defeat themselves is with the thoughts they think and the words they speak. I have seen it repeatedly with people, including myself. I began changing my thoughts and words years ago, thanks to my wonderful husband. It took time, but I have mostly mastered this component of health. Like Brennan Manning, "I began loving myself into a fresh way of thinking," because I understood I was worth it.

Let me give you an outstanding example of how your thoughts affect your health. My husband and I were in a car accident in 2006. I had been in several prior car accidents in my life, including a terrible head-on collision in college, and a thirteen-car pileup on I-75 in Atlanta when my kids were young. Unfortunately, in those times I did not know about chiropractic and other treatment modalities. As a result, I have some back and neck issues and have degenerating vertebrae in my neck. When this accident occurred in 2006, it really exacerbated my neck issues, and I spent almost a year in chronic pain. Finally, after ten months of misery, I made a choice to change the narrative I was telling myself. I took my focus off my pain and started living again. Although the pain was still there, changing my focus and the words I spoke (I stopped talking about the pain to myself or others far too much), helped me feel better. Little by little, my neck got better. It was all because I changed my thoughts and words. I started speaking about health instead of pain. I focused on my passion and purpose instead of wallowing in self-pity. It was such an eye opener to me about the power of my thoughts and words. They literally have the power of life and death.

As I've become more aware of how thoughts influence how we feel, I observe how often people use their thoughts and words to defeat themselves. Claiming illnesses as "mine" is one way. You know how it goes, "Oh 'my' allergies are acting up." Or "Today 'my' arthritis is really bothering me." I suggest that if you don't claim such things as yours, that you change the narrative. They aren't yours. Send them back! Don't receive them as yours. If you must talk about whatever is challenging you, you could use lingo like this instead: "I'm currently being challenged with a bit of allergies (arthritis, etc.), but I'm getting better as we speak." No longer take ownership of those challenges. Look at them as minor inconveniences and seek to find out how you can take part in the healing process. It begins with changing your thoughts and words, which will then change your feelings, your actions, and ultimately your results. I suggest you spend time visualizing a healthy body. So often we think we must see it to believe it—but I'm suggesting you must believe it to see it.

I have used affirmations often in my life. My health is one area I have benefited from affirmations. A great affirmation to say and put up around your house, car, etc., is, "I am healthy, vibrant, and fit! Every cell in my body functions perfectly." During challenging times with my back, I have recited that affirmation over and over while taking a bike ride or walking or doing some other mindless activity. Notice I attached the affirmation to my exercise routine, which also ultimately helped my back. When you put something in your subconscious enough, you believe it and make it a reality. I will talk more about affirmations later in the chapter.

We have conscious thoughts of which we are aware, and subconscious thoughts of which we are unaware. We don't feel our thoughts at the subconscious level. There is one way to know what you believe at the subconscious level. Look at your results.

Going back to our TFAR acronym, you can trace your results back to your thoughts and many times, your subconscious thoughts. Results never lie. Therefore, if you believe deep down that you don't deserve to be healthy, you will make unhealthy choices that manifest illness. It's what you believe at the subconscious level, and the subconscious must always be right.

According to a 2005 National Science Foundation article based on research about human thoughts per day, the average person has around 12,000 to 60,000 thoughts per day. Apparently, research has shown that on average about eighty percent of those thoughts are negative, and a large percentage are repetitive from the day before.[115] We think the same thoughts repeatedly, and about eighty percent of them are negative. Ugh! No wonder we experience poor results.

"Words kill, words give life; they're either poison or fruit—you choose."

Proverbs 18:21, MSG

YOUR DNA IS NOT YOUR DESTINY!

To show how your thoughts, positively or negatively, affect your health, think about the "placebo" effect. I'm sure you are aware of this phenomenon. They found that when people are given a placebo—such as sugar pills, fake surgeries, saline injections—they recover from eighteen to eighty percent of the time.

In contrast, the "nocebo" effect shows how negative beliefs—fear, anxiety, or learned victimhood—affect your health. I have seen families unknowingly propagate in their kids' minds their entire

---

[115] https://siobhankukolic.com/the-average-person-has-between-12000-and-60000-thoughts-per-day/

lives this notion that certain illnesses run in their family. They are truly operating from a good place thinking they are warning their kids so they can protect them, when in fact they are constantly planting the seeds of the diseases in their kids' minds. It is no surprise then when those kids become adults that they end up with those same illnesses. They have subconsciously believed almost their entire lives that the illnesses were their destiny, and so there it is. It saddens me more than I can say. Women even have prophylactic mastectomies because breast cancer "runs" in their family. How sad to buy into that kind of fear. What people don't realize is that if you have the lifestyle, exposure to toxins, subconscious beliefs, or whatever else causes cancer, you will get cancer somewhere in the body, even if you don't have breasts. It can just happen somewhere else.

I am also opposed to all the new tests that check you for genetic predispositions to all manner of disease. I know doctors often do these tests to motivate people to make lifestyle changes to prevent the disease, but I believe that it just plants seeds in their minds that can cause them to manifest the specific disease in their lives. The mind is a powerful thing.

My mom lived to ninety in fairly good shape until the last few years. She passed away in 2011 a couple of months after her ninetieth birthday. A few years before she passed away, we found out she had breast cancer. She apparently got a mammogram soon after her only sister died of breast cancer in 1990, and it showed something suspicious. My mom never went back to follow up on that suspicious place, and never went back to the gynecologist. She loathed hospitals and wanted to avoid the terrible path of treatment my sweet aunt went through. My mother did not die of breast cancer. She had it when she died, but it did not kill her. I'm convinced that her avoiding medical treatment for that helped keep her alive for over twenty years longer. She was also proactive and did healthy things I recommended, like juicing, taking Barley Green, and then taking Juice Plus+ for years.

After Mom admitted to us that she had some breast tumors, she agreed to go get a biopsy. I did not suggest for her to see the oncologist. I knew she would not do the treatments they would suggest, and going through a painful biopsy was pointless, in my opinion. But my siblings convinced her otherwise because they wanted to know if it was "genetic." I told them clearly that I was opting out of knowing those results (yes, they thought I was crazy, but it seems I'm the unicorn in my family). I know the power of the mind and as I told them, I was already doing everything I knew to prevent breast cancer (eating a whole-food vegan diet, exercise, etc.). I had also taught my daughter the same principles. I did not want the idea of a genetic predisposition in my head because of how powerful beliefs are in determining outcomes. It turns out mom's cancer was not genetic. As I mentioned earlier, even if they considered it genetic, I believe my lifestyle determines whether I turn those genes on or off, and I would not get breast cancer. Remember, your genes are not your destiny, *unless* you believe they are.

Now I am not suggesting you don't get various exams such as colonoscopies or breast thermograms (my choice over mammograms) to catch cancer early on. I'm suggesting the genetic tests may not be ideal because they plant seeds in your mind that can easily grow and become self-fulfilling prophecies. Instead, I recommend adopting the principles in this book to prevent most all diseases, without planting negative seeds in your mind from those tests. Remember, begin with the end in mind. Whether you have genetic predispositions to certain things or not, you have the power to turn on or off your genes! That has been proven repeatedly in scientific studies (read *The China Study* by T. Colin Campbell, PHD).

In summary, you must reprogram your thoughts and your words to make sure they are true, noble, pure, lovely, and praiseworthy (Phil 4:8). I believe we have the mind of our Creator, which means we get to think brilliantly. Anytime we are thinking negatively about ourselves and others, we are not thinking brilliantly.

If you want to change the results you are getting in your life, you must change your thoughts. Start thinking thoughts of health, vitality, peace, and joy. Your results will change. Stop using negative thoughts and words against yourself. Stop claiming illnesses as your own. Start speaking life over yourself and others. Then you will put in the work to make those pure and lovely thoughts a reality. It's almost like magic.

> "Genes may start the job but they don't finish it. The far more important question we should ask is 'what controls the expression of genes that lead to health and disease events?' Experimental and extensively published research over several decades has long convinced me that nutrition primarily provides this control."
>
> T. Colin Campbell, PhD

WHY ARE YOU HERE?

Mark Twain said, "The two most important days in your life are the day you are born, and the day you find out why." When I do health talks, I often start out by asking people to raise their hands if they believe they are on this planet for a reason. Almost everyone raises their hand. I then ask them to keep their hand raised if they know what their purpose is. Sadly, the large majority put their hand down. The reason I start my talks this way is because I believe that knowing your purpose for being on this planet is a key component to your health. You may scratch your head asking why I think that. The reason I believe that is that after working with people for years, helping them adopt a healthy lifestyle, those who connect with a personal purpose are better, by far, at practicing self-care than those who don't connect with their purpose.

Your purpose is your primary gift to the world. It is where your deep sadness connects with someone else's deep need. Figuring out what your purpose is can be a challenge, because it requires you to be still and do some praying and soul searching. For whatever reason, many people avoid it. I think there are several reasons that people avoid figuring out their purpose: they don't believe they are worthy of a calling, they are subconsciously fearful of digging deep within, they have past hurts that caused them to lose hope, they are too busy to figure it out (often working a job they are unsatisfied in), and they find it hard to figure out. No matter your age, I encourage you to do the work to figure out the reason you are still on this planet, no matter how young or old you are. You are still here, which means you still have a reason to be here. Your life will be so much more meaningful when you connect with your unique purpose. And I suggest you will take better care of yourself because it will motivate you to fulfill that purpose.

PURPOSE FINDER EXERCISE

Have the courage to listen to your heart and intuition. They somehow already know what you truly want to become."

Steve Jobs

Here is a purpose finder exercise to help you zone in on why you are here. I encourage you to put the effort and time in this process. It will be worth it. Answer the following questions honestly. Answer with your heart. Don't worry about what others will think. This is about you right now. It's about what is deep within you. Go with your gut response.

- When do I feel most joyful, alive, and fulfilled?

_____

_____

_____

- What natural talents and interests do I have?

_____

_____

_____

- What do I love doing?

_____

_____

_____

- What am I passionate about?

_____

_____

_____

- What do people compliment me on?

_____

_____

_____

- If I could make a difference in any area/issue/problem, what would it be? (i.e., human trafficking, world hunger, child abuse, animal abuse, etc.)

_____

_____

_____

- If I knew I couldn't fail, what would I do with my life?

_____

_____

_____

- Based on my answers above, what is my purpose in 2-3 sentences?

_____

_____

_____

I provide my purpose statement as an example: "My purpose is to be a beacon of light guiding people to the truth that eliminates suffering, and brings vitality in body, soul and spirit."

Now that you know your purpose, I hope it will motivate you to take care of yourself so you can fulfill that purpose! The world needs you to shine. Playing small benefits no one! I believe you can accomplish great things, all while staying humble. If you'd like help with breaking down your purpose into actionable goals, check out our Flourish program at PureLightHealth.com.

I believe your purpose changes and morphs over time. When I was raising kids, that was my primary purpose. And it is one of the most noble things I have ever done. Now that I'm a grand-mother (did I mention how much I love being a grandma?), part of my purpose is playing a major role in my grandkid's lives. You can keep the right priorities in life all while fulfilling your purpose. My priorities are—God first, my family second, and then my mission/business. When I'm asked to do some-thing, I filter it through these priorities. That means I will never be a workaholic, because work is third on my list. Being a workaholic requires far too much time away from my top two priorities. It is a delicate balance that takes time to figure out, but it's worth doing. Working towards your purpose, all while keeping the right priorities, will bring you satisfaction and joy, and dare I say make you healthier!

"If purpose were a pill, it would be a blockbuster drug. People who know their sense of purpose live about eight years longer than people who are rudderless."

Dan Buettner

BREAK YOUR PURPOSE INTO SMART GOALS

Once you know your purpose, it's important to establish some goals to move you in the right direction towards fulfilling it. I have used the SMART process for goal setting for many years with success. I encourage you to use this process to create some health/lifestyle goals, as being in good health is essen-tial to you fulfilling your purpose. Establishing goals is vital to getting where you want to go. Setting SMART goals is begin-ning with the end in mind, as I discussed earlier. If you don't set goals, you might end up somewhere you don't want to be. When you start out on a vacation, you know where you want to go, correct? Therefore, you have a map on how to get there, or a plane ticket with the right destination booked. Having goals is just like that. It's the map to help you fulfill your purpose. Here are the details of the SMART process:

- **Specific**: Your goals must be specific to be terrific! You need to know specifically what you want to accomplish. As an example, you can't just say, "I want to lose weight." Instead, you might say, "I want to achieve my ideal weight of _____ pounds."

- **Measurable**: Your goals also need to be measurable. Otherwise, your subconscious mind can't act if it doesn't know what to grab onto. A measurable goal for the above example would be, "I will eat 100% whole plant foods, exercise 5 days per week for 30 minutes, and achieve my ideal weight of _____ pounds."

- **Attainable**: Your goal must be attainable to be realistic. For example, losing 20 pounds in 6 months is attainable. Losing 300 pounds in 6 months is not attainable, nor would it be healthy. You know something is attainable if it makes it in your calendar. Putting 30 minutes a day for 5 days per week of exercise in your calendar is attainable. Exercising for 8 hours per day, 7 days per week, is not attainable.

- **Relevant**: The goal must apply to you. It must be something you want deep-down, not something someone else wants for you. The relevancy factor is the why for setting the goal. For this example, the relevancy could be this, "Eating healthy, exercising, and achieving my ideal weight will give me the confidence I need and desperately want to be a good example to my loved ones. It will allow me to influence the people I care most about with my example."

- **Timely**: For goals to be meaningful, you must establish a time frame to accomplish them; otherwise, there will always be excuses to do something else, and put your goal off. In this case, "I will eat a whole-food plant-based diet, exercise, and achieve my ideal weight of _____ pounds within 6 months, starting on January 1, 2022, which will help me have more energy and be a good example for my loved ones." You then take that six-month goal and break it down to monthly, weekly, and daily goals. Most importantly, you get the actions in your calendar to guarantee your success. The most important part of goal setting is determining the actions that will get you to your destination.

IT'S YOUR TURN—SET YOUR SMART HEALTH GOAL

If you knew you couldn't fail, what health goal would you like to accomplish in 90 days that meets these criteria?

Specific:

_____

_____

Measurable:

_____

_____

Attainable:

_____

_____

Relevant:

_____

_____

Timely:

_____

_____

State your 90-day goal in 1-2 sentences:

_____

_____

Congratulations! You have taken a huge first step towards a more vibrant, happier you! As Georgia O'Keefe said, "You get whatever accomplishment you are willing to declare." I work with people helping them understand themselves and others better using LifeThrive's unique system that looks at behaviors (aka personality) and mindsets (aka priorities). I've found these assessments invaluable in helping to set goals in accordance with how you are uniquely designed, making the process much more effective and efficient. If you are interested in finding out more, check out my Flourish program at www.PureLightHealth.com/flourish or go to www.LifeThrive.com to take one of their free assessments. Mention my name as to who referred you!

FINDING FAITH THAT FREES

"I believe in God the Father
Almighty Maker of Heaven and Maker of Earth
And in Jesus Christ His only begotten Son our Lord
I believe in the Holy Spirit
One Holy Church
The communion of saints
The forgiveness of sin
I believe in the resurrection
I believe in a life that never ends
And I believe what I believe is what makes me what I am

I did not make it, no it is making me
I did not make it, no it is making me
I said I did not make it, no it is making me
It is the very truth of God and not the invention of any man"[116]

I have had a spiritual hunger for as long as I can remember. As a child, I remember being drawn to spiritual things. I grew up Roman Catholic in the small town of Elizabethtown, Kentucky. We went to church every week, and I spent the first six years of grade school and my Junior year in high school attending Catholic schools.

My faith journey has not been a smooth ride for sure, as I'm sure most people can relate to. It has had many ups and downs, and I have had lots of crises of faith over the years. My first crisis of faith happened on November 6, 1968. I had just celebrated my eleventh birthday twelve days earlier. I was walking home one crisp November afternoon thinking about some things I wanted to try with my hair when I got home, some new style I had heard about or something. I was excited to get home and do my hair experiment. However, three blocks from home my mom's best friend, Aunt Martha, stopped me. She asked me to come into their house instead of going home because my brother Bobby had been in a car accident that day. She also summoned my younger brother, John, similarly on his walk home. Later that evening, after we had eaten dinner, a moment I will never forget happened. John and I were playing upstairs with our "cousins" when Aunt Martha called us downstairs into the living room. When we walked in there, the parish priest was with my sister Nancy and clearly, they were the bearers of bad news. They informed us that our older brother Bobby, then eighteen, had not survived the auto accident. He was gone! It was a horrible moment in my life that forever changed me. Obviously, God did not exist as I had prayed many nights for Him to protect my

---

[116] Rich Mullins, D. Beaker, (1993). "Creed", *A Liturgy, A Legacy & A Ragamuffin Band*. Retrieved from https://www.azlyrics.com/lyrics/richmullins/creed.html

family, and He had not. Therefore, in my eleven-year-old mind, He must not be real!

After we were told the bad news, my sister tried to comfort us. I remember running off when they told us—I could not face the truth. My sister took us home to see our parents. I remember walking into our home filled with people. My parents were in the den area with a bunch of other people, and I remember going over to my mom and hugging her and crying. Fear racked my little body, and to this day, I shake when my brother's death comes up in a conversation with my family. My older siblings have filled me in on the back-story of that day in November of 1968, when my brother clung to life, only to have it slip away a few hours later. It was not a happy day in the Nusz family, or our small community. It was one that affected every member of our family profoundly, especially my parents. My parents turned to alcohol to help soothe the hurt, which left me feeling "less than." There were times I wanted to say, "But I'm still here," not understanding the intense pain a parent feels losing a child. I think subconsciously I believed I was not good enough since I could not ease their pain. Each time they chose alcohol reinforced that belief in my mind. Wasn't I good enough to make them not want to drink? Oh, the toxic beliefs we develop as children that follow us through life, until we confront them and detoxify and replace them with healthy, God thoughts! I will share in a bit how God would later speak to me about that experience and gradually reprogram my thinking.

My brother's auto accident and death on November 6, 1968, was a Kairos (defining) moment in my life, and it taught me several lessons that carry with me today. Foremost, I recognized life can change on a dime. That morning was like every other morning in my household. We all busily got ready for our days, had breakfast, and took off in different directions. We said goodbye in the usual manner and thought nothing special about that goodbye. It was like every other one, except it wasn't. It was the last goodbye with Bobby, but none of us, including him, were aware that it would be the last. We would have lingered longer had we only known.

I also learned that day that our decisions have ripple effects and affect not only us. His poor decision to get in a car with other college freshman that day and travel forty-five minutes to buy alcohol and drink it while driving affected us all (he was not the driver). It rocked every one of our lives profoundly and robbed him of his at the young age of 18! Both my parents ended up with bleeding ulcers within a year of that day, my mom sooner than my dad. My mom ended up having one-third of her stomach cut out in a risky surgery that could have taken her life. I remember being woken up in the night and told that she made it through the surgery. Whew, what a relief for an eleven-year-old who had only months before lost her big brother. I was a big-time momma's girl, and the thought of losing her was so scary!

The biggest lesson I learned that day was that life was precious, and we needed to enjoy every moment to the fullest. None of us are promised tomorrow so, carpe diem, seize this day. We may not have tomorrow! I learned that our loved ones might not be around tomorrow, so enjoy every second you have with them today. Take nothing for granted! Seize every moment you have with those you care about, so there are no regrets. This lesson guides my priorities in life. Next to God, my loved ones are second, and that is why spending time with them takes precedence in my schedule. I will drop most everything to spend time with loved ones. It is why I left corporate America to pursue my own business. I needed to dictate my time. To me, time is abundantly more important than money. Of course, one needs money to own your time, but there are many ways to simplify your life to spend it doing what's important. John Robbins in *The New Good Life* said, "As to the path to happiness and the good life, Thomas Jefferson reminded us that, 'It is neither wealth nor splendor, but tranquility and occupation which give happiness.'"[117]

GET BACK UP AGAIN

A few of the lyrics from the song "Get Back Up Again" (Sung by Anna Kendrick in the popular kid's movie, Trolls), summarize my spiritual journey over the years. They are:

"Hey! I'm not giving up today.
There's nothing getting in my way.
And if you knock-knock me over,
I will get back up again.
Oh, and if something goes a little wrong,
Well, you can go ahead and bring it on,
'Cause if you knock-knock me over,
I will get back up again.
What if it's all a big mistake?
What if it's more than I can take?
No, I can't think that way.
'Cause I know that I'm really-really-really gonna be okay."[118]

My granddaughter Juliette, when she was four years old, was so great at singing this when she took a little tumble (most of the time anyway). She would pop back up singing this song. It makes me smile and gives me a glorious reminder on how I want to live my life. Over the years my faith has taken many tumbles, but I have always popped back up again. At times it was days or weeks or months or even years (as was the case

[117] John Robbins, *The New Good Life: Living Better Than Ever in an Age of Less*, Kindle edition, (Ballantine Books, 2010), loc 1184

[118] Benj Pasek, Justin Noble Paul, (2016). "Get Back Up Again", *Trolls (Original Motion Picture Soundtrack)*. Universal Music Publishing Group. Retrieved from https://www.lyrics.com/lyric/33271608/Anna+Kendrick/Get+Back+Up+Again

after my brother died) until I got back up again, but I eventually realized that I'd rather do life believing in a higher power than not. God has proven Himself to me so many times that not believing God exists isn't an option for me. I know God exists. You can't convince me otherwise. I haven't always had such a rock-solid belief. It's been sixty-four years developing. My time period between falling and getting back up on the faith "saddle" is typically very short now. Thankfully!

When my brother died in 1968, it knocked me off that saddle. I just could not wrap my mind around God allowing Bobby to die. I mean, if He could not protect my brother when I had prayed so diligently most nights, what good was He anyway? Many of my crises of faith came when God did not answer my prayer the way I wanted, as I'm sure most of us can attest to. That version of God is more of a genie in a bottle. God should grant my every wish, right? Imagine if that was the case and every person on the planet got their wishes granted, every time. Do you think there might be some conflicting things going on? Yea, I'm pretty sure there would be.

What I later learned was that God gave humans the one thing that He gave no other creature on this planet, the power to choose. He gave *us* the power to choose. Think about that! No other creature has that power but us. Wow! He has not revoked that gift since the beginning of creation. One of our choices is the choice to believe, love, and follow Him, or not. He does not force Himself on us. Who wants forced love anyway? We all deep down want love that is given freely by the giver, right?

I realized that truth—that we have the God-given power to choose—in another Kairos moment of my faith journey. One Saturday in 1993, I spent all afternoon reading a book that forever changed my life. The title of the book is *The Greatest Miracle in The World* by Og Mandino. I read that book and wept. God used it to whisper His love into my spirit that day, and I have never been the same. The message of the book, told in only a way that Og can tell, is that we are God's greatest miracle. It contains in it "The God Memorandum" which I firmly believe was given to Og by an angel. If you haven't read that book and the sequel titled *Return of the Ragpicker*, please do yourself a favor and read them as soon as you finish this book. I believe they will change your life as they did mine!

An excerpt from "The God Memorandum": "You were a marvel to behold, and I was pleased. I gave you this world and dominion over it. Then, to enable you to reach your full potential I placed my hand upon you, once more, and endowed you with powers unknown to any other creature in the universe, even unto this day. I gave you the power to think. I gave you the power to love. I gave you the power to will. I gave you the power to laugh. I gave you the power to imagine. I gave you the power to create. I gave you the power to plan. I gave you the power to speak. I gave you the power to pray. My pride in you knew no bounds. You were my ultimate creation, my greatest miracle. A complete living being. One who can adjust to any climate, any hardship, any challenge. One who can manage his own destiny without any interference from me. One who can translate a sensation or perception, not by instinct, but by thought and deliberation into whatever action is best for him(her)self and all humanity. Thus, we come to the fourth law of success and happiness... for I gave you one more power, a power so great that not even my angels possess it. I gave you... the power to choose."[119]

So many people refuse to believe that there is a god because of one argument. An argument you have probably used if you don't believe in a Creator. I have used it before. Most people do at some point. The argument is this: there cannot possibly be a god because bad things happen to good people. If there was a god, he would not allow such unfairness to happen. I wrestled with this so many times in my life. There is such horror and evil that often seems to prevail in our world. Human trafficking,

---

[119]   Og Mandino, *The Greatest Miracle in the World*, (Bantam, 1983)

animal torture, sexual assaults, greediness, meanness, bullying, and on and on it goes. How can God sit back and allow such horror? One reason—He gave us the power to choose, and He will not take that power away from us.

Think about a world where God controlled every one of us. What do you think it would be like? I suppose we would all be little robots walking around. Everything would be wonderful and blissful all day every day. How do you think that would be? If there were never cloudy days, would you appreciate the sun? If no challenges ever existed in your life, would you grow? Would you appreciate the good times as much if you had no bad times to compare them to? I know I would not! Most of the motivation in my life to grow and improve has been born out of pain, heartache, and challenges. When I'm on the mountaintop, when everything is going great, I just don't feel that I need God as much. I know I need Him all the time, but I do not *feel* the urgency to connect with Him as much on the mountaintop. It's in the valleys of life where I am drawn to the Creator and forced to face my own demons. I don't believe God ever causes harm. He is love—pure agape love that never fails. We are the creators of harm, malice, and anything less than good. Not God! He allows us to do bad things because He decided when He created the world that He would give us free will. It is up to us to be the change we wish to see in the world, to be a force for good, to bring about peace, and to be an accurate representation of our God, which would ultimately draw people to Him.

LORD SAVE ME FROM YOUR FOLLOWERS

As I mentioned, I remember having a hunger for God since I was a child. Unfortunately, several times I got off the faith saddle because of people who called themselves Christians. The way they represented God made me not want to believe. I confused them and their actions with God, and deemed that if He was like "them," then I would do better off without Him. It was really my fault because I made the mistake of looking to people versus seeing who God was for me. I have seen this bumper sticker on people's cars and chuckled because I have felt the same way: "Lord save me from Your followers." I'm quite sure people have said that about me at times, especially when I'm being judgmental or narcissistic.

My experience being raised Catholic was that God was like this mean dude in the sky holding a baseball bat, ready to whack us each time we messed up. I'm not sure why I thought that, but I did. I go back to a Catholic mass now and the liturgy really does not imply this notion. Like many denominations, there can be a "works" mentality in the Catholic faith. If you say enough Hail Mary's or Our Father's, go to confession enough, or give enough money, then you will be right with God. My first church experience outside of the Catholic faith as an adult perpetuated this works-mentality. It was probably even more prevalent there than in Catholicism. I'm not suggesting that we don't serve where God plants us. I'm suggesting that we can never equate how much we do or don't do with our salvation. Our salvation results from believing and professing that Jesus is the one and only Messiah (Savior). Period!

One of the precious men God brought in our lives several years ago after we experienced some serious hurts by Christians (a topic for another day), was an ex-missionary who had such a heart for people. I remember him saying, "When you wake up in the morning there is nothing you can do to make God love you anymore. And there is nothing you can do to make God love you any less." Bam—another Kairos moment in my life and spiritual journey. It set me free in so many ways. What is interesting is that when you really get that message—that God loves you unconditionally no matter what you do, or don't do—then love drives you to "do" more to honor and serve Him. I believe that people in many churches "do" more because they feel they must, to gain God's approval. Sadly, they do not understand that God loves them because of who He is, not because of anything they do. Often what we really need to do is just "be."

I realized that after my years being raised Roman Catholic, combined with several years in a non-denominational Christian church, that I did not understand what God's grace was, let alone know how to receive it freely. Thus, I began a quest to learn about and understand to my very core what the grace of God is. I started reading books like *The Ragamuffin Gospel* by Brennan Manning, *The Shack* by William Paul Young, and *What's So Amazing About Grace* by Phillip Yancey. I cannot even express in words the joy I felt learning God is a god of love and grace. He loves me—PERIOD! I don't have to do anything or be anything for Him to love me. He loves me because He is God, and He is LOVE! Period, end of discussion. Merriam-Webster's Dictionary defines grace as: "unmerited (not adequately earned or deserved) divine assistance given humans for their regeneration or sanctification; approval, favor."[120] I say grace is undeserved favor. I have done nothing to deserve God's favor, and honestly, I have done many things in my life to disqualify me from it. But alas, He gives it to me anyway. And He will give it to you as well. Thankfully!

My negative experiences with God's followers tempted me, like many, to abandon my faith. I dealt with confusion and blurring the lines between God and people. I had to pull away and experience for myself who God really was for me. I was not willing to go through life without faith. This life has too many challenges and pain to do it without divine guidance and comfort. I had spent lots of years trying to do it alone, and that was no longer an option I would consider. I put God to the test, and He came through time and time again. Has He answered every prayer I have prayed the way I wanted, and done everything I wanted Him to do? Heck no! Has He taken away every hurt I have felt or challenge I have faced? Nope. But I have learned that God is always with me, even, and especially when I'm hurting.

---

[120] https://www.merriam-webster.com/dictionary/grace

This was most clear to me after my mom died. I had a really hard time with her death. Growing up, I was a momma's girl, and I got the honor of spending a lot of time with her over the years before her passing. I grieved deeply to where I would cry uncontrollably for hours on end. I felt as if I could not breathe; the pain was so strong. I cried out to God during those moments of intense grief, and I can tell you this based on my experience: He did NOT take the pain away. What He did was enable me to get through it. I knew He was there in the darkness. He provided the "ministry of presence" to me in my toughest moments, and I always knew that I would get through it. The bottom line is that grief hurts, a lot, but when you grieve (and we all will in our lives), cry out to the Lord, and I believe He will provide you with that life-saving ministry of presence that will get you through the darkest days. Test Him and see. Just say, "Jesus, help!" That's all you need to do. He will never leave you nor forsake you! (Deut 4:31) Trust Him in that!

RUTHLESS TRUST

Thanks to my brother being killed in a car accident when I was eleven, my biggest fear when I had my own kids was that something would happen to them. I knew this fear was there, but I did not verbalize it. I tried willing and praying it away, but it still lingered (and still does to a lesser extent). My son Enrique called me on it when he was a teenager, and I was being perhaps stricter than I needed to be with him (he liked to push the boundaries). I still remember the moment standing in his room when he said to me, "Mom, you've got to stop treating me this way just because your brother died. I'm not him." Wow, from the mouth of babes! God used my kids to speak into my life on many, many occasions. This was another Kairos moment. I knew I had to face this fear head on and deal with it. About that time, I found a book by Brennan Manning titled *Ruthless Trust*, that helped set me free (mostly) of this fear.[121] After reading that book, I declared to the Lord, "I choose to ruthlessly trust you, EVEN if one of my children dies." Gulp!

I have several close friends who have lost children, which exacerbated my fear of losing a child. One of the most influential people in my life is Ramona. She is one of the lifeboats God sent me! She has been a spiritual mom to me for years, and of course one of my best friends. When I first met Ramona and became friends with her, she had already lost her son Brian quite a few years before. He was eighteen and died in a car accident like my brother. Ramona traveled often and gave her amazing testimony to Christian women's clubs of how God got her through that excruciatingly painful experience. Her testimony touched me powerfully each time I heard it. Then the unthinkable happened in December of 2004. Ramona lost her only daughter Pam in the same way she lost Brian, in a car accident. I was absolutely in shock when I got the call that night from Ramona's only remaining child, Wayne. I rushed over to her house, packed with friends, and cried with her and all the others who were there. I will never forget the look in that beautiful woman's eyes in the limo at the graveyard after Pam's service. It was a look like I have never seen before or since. It was a look of utter desperation and sorrow. That look was raw, and it touched me deeply. All I could think was that I wanted to do anything and everything I could to ease her pain and comfort her. But how? I called my good friend and spiritual mentor, Dean, with many questions. He gave wise counsel and said the only thing that I could do was to offer the "ministry of presence." He explained that just being there, listening, hugging when needed, crying, understanding, and not trying to offer solutions (there are none), is what my friend most needed. I have learned it is the only thing any of us can offer to someone suffering. And it is enough.

---

[121]   Brennan Manning, *Ruthless Trust: The Ragamuffin's Path to God*, (Harper Collins, 2009)

I saw Ramona at least every week, and I witnessed a slow miracle occur in her and her precious husband, Bill. I saw God see them through. It is my opinion that there are three things that heal grief: a strong faith, people to provide the ministry of presence, and time. Does my friend still miss her daughter these years later? I know she does. She will until the day she is reunited with both of her kids, and now her husband of 63 years. But I have witnessed a woman who loves and empathizes like no one else I know. No matter how "shallow" or large my pain or trials, she is always there for me. She encourages and prays. She reassures me that God has not forgotten me, and that He is still there, even though I may not feel Him. Ramona's faith gives me hope and makes me want to have stronger faith. She and Bill took two unthinkable tragedies in their lives and allowed God to turn them around for good. They impacted so many people with their example of "faith no matter what." I have told Ramona that I know her mansion is going to be HUGE in Heaven, and I'm hoping I get to visit often.

I have had other friends who have lost children, some I have spent a good bit of time with (although none as much as Ramona) after their loss, and others not as much. One day I was grieving for my friend who lost her two-year-old son to drowning and I asked God, "Why do I have so many friends who have lost children? It's so hard seeing them suffer so much." And as sure as I'm sitting here today, I heard in my spirit God tell me, "So you would know how deeply moms hurt after losing children, and you would finally understand that your parents loved you. They were just hurting so bad after your brother's death that they could not give you what you needed. It was not about you! It was about their deep pain. They loved you!" I wept and wept when He revealed that to me. That revelation was the healing balm I needed. Another Kairos moment in my life! God wastes no experiences in your life and will use them for your good if you allow Him.

Finding faith that frees—I have searched many years to find a faith that frees me from myself, from my demons, from the need for the approval of people, and from the wounds of my past. Through searching and continuing to search, I have found this faith that truly frees. I assure you the faith I searched for and found was born out of my trials and pain; it did not come during the mountaintop experiences in my life. My pain drove me to search for meaning beyond myself. God has spoken to me in so many ways—mostly through nature and people. It is beyond me how people can experience a sunset or sunrise, a beautiful baby smiling, the tenderness of a kiss from a loved one, and many other things without believing there is something bigger and beyond us. I don't pretend to understand everything about God, and I am not a Biblical scholar, but I have a deep desire to know Him more with each passing day. The Creator of the universe speaks to my spirit and helps me with this journey called life. He will help you too!

Do you think God stopped communicating with people with the last words of the Bible? I don't! First, that makes no sense (I'm a very logical person, hence I used to be an accountant), and secondly, I have had too many actual experiences where God spoke to my spirit. I love what my friend Kathrine Lee says, "Come on, you just can't make this stuff up!" I could tell you story after story of how God has orchestrated things in my life that I could not make up. I believe there are no coincidences in life. All things happen for a reason, and although I don't believe God causes bad things to happen, I believe as Graham Cooke says, "God allows in His wisdom what He could easily prevent with His power." I also believe that there are some things we just won't understand this side of Heaven. That is where faith comes in.

What if I and the multitude of people who believe in the Creator of the universe are wrong and there is no god? I have lost nothing believing, and only gained heaven on Earth. My faith frees me to believe that God loves me no matter what, and that His plans for me are good. Although I experience pain, challenges, and doubt in this world, I choose to receive Jesus' peace that surpasses understanding. As Ramona taught me, I trust the one who holds my future when I don't know what my future holds. I choose to have ruthless trust that no matter what happens to me, that God will see me through. I choose to believe, as my friend Gigi did, that "in the eye of the storm, that God remains in control (not that He controls us or our circumstances). I choose to believe that in the middle of the war, that He will guard my soul. He alone is my anchor when my sails are torn." (From "The Eye of the Storm" (Lyrics, 2015) sung by Ryan Stevenson)[122]

As Rich's song says in the beginning of this section, it's not the invention of any man, but the very truth of God. Jesus Christ summarized it when He said, "Love the Lord your God with all your heart and with all your soul and with all your mind."[123] And, "Love your neighbor as yourself."[124] Did you catch that? He said love your neighbor *as* yourself, which implies you must first love yourself. Oh, I could go on and on regarding how we can't even love ourselves because of all the lies we have bought over the years, but we will save that for another book. He said to love our neighbor, not if they are like us, if we agree with them, if we are of the same political party, or if we like them. He said to love them. If every person on the planet practiced these three things: love God, love self, and love others, our world would be peaceful and full of bliss. There would be no wars, greed, corruption, violence, or hatred. All would be love!

Finding faith that frees, by practicing these three things Jesus taught, is one foundation of health. Will you embrace this foundation and experience heaven on earth? I hope you will! This

---

[122] Ryan Stevenson, *The Eye of the Storm* lyrics, https://www.lyrics.com/track/32771296/Ryan+Stevenson/Eye+of+the+Storm

[123] Matthew 22:37, NIV

[124] Matthew 22:39, NIV

kind of faith gets me through life—the good, the bad, the beautiful, and the ugly. It helps me get up every day with a heart of gratitude, no matter what I'm going through! It helps me forgive those who hurt me, love the unlovable, persist when I want to quit, and be a person of integrity. It helps me to love myself by practicing self-care. It helps me know that "except for God, there go I" when I see so many angry, judgmental, depressed, and unhealthy people. My desire, as Mahatma Gandhi taught, is to be the change I wish to see in the world. I can only do that with the help of Almighty God. In and of myself, I simply can't.

I encourage you to embrace the Creator of the universe. He loves you beyond what you can even imagine. Simply reach out and grab His hand. I believe it's outstretched to you! Let go of holding people up as God, and their actions as His. Be willing to ask questions of Him and allow Him to answer in a way that only He can. Seek and you shall find! Commit to the process of spiritual growth so you can experience Heaven on Earth. Spiritual health is a component to vitality and health. Without it, there is no wholeness. With it, all things are possible to those who believe! I will pray for you! And if you'd like an impactful, fun way to learn more about Jesus, I recommend *The Chosen* TV series.[125]

"I was one way and now I am completely different, and the thing that happened in between, was Him."

Mary Magdalene in The Chosen

---

[125]   https://watch.angelstudios.com/thechosen

MOVE YOUR BODY

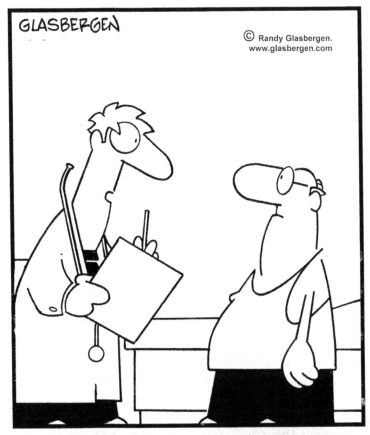

GLASBERGEN

© Randy Glasbergen.
www.glasbergen.com

"What fits your busy schedule better,
exercising one hour a day or being
dead 24 hours a day?"

I know you know how important movement is in a healthy lifestyle, but it bears repeating. To live in peak health, it is imperative to move your body daily. And I don't mean just getting up
and walking to the pantry to get more chips and salsa while you
are watching TV at night. I am talking about moving as part of
your daily life. Exercise is an absolute must for all your life. The
moment you stop moving, you stagnate, and decline.

I saw an obvious example of this with my mom. My mom was always an active woman. She had seven children so I'm sure she got plenty of exercise in her younger years taking care of all of us. But she also loved playing tennis and started playing tennis after we were all gone from the house. She loved to walk as well and at times could out-walk me in her later years. She continued batting a tennis ball and walking the hills of Kentucky and Southern Indiana until she was about eighty-eight years old. She had a little heart scare at that age and was afraid to go out and walk after it. Despite my sister Karen (whose property Mom lived on) urging her to exercise, she rarely did it after her episode. I saw my vibrant mom, who could walk up steep hills, go downhill quickly once she stopped moving. She became feeble in no time because of her lack of movement. I vowed then that I would stay active my whole life, no matter what!

Movement is one habit of centenarians in the blue zones that is a key to their longevity and quality of life. As I mentioned, the blue zones are the areas in the world that have the longest-lived people who live disability-free. One of the nine blue zones' lessons is to move naturally each day. It's not so much about having a purposeful exercise regime as it is to incorporate movement into your daily life. Here is what www.bluezones.com says about movement: "The world's longest-lived people don't pump iron, run marathons, or join gyms. Instead, they live in environments that constantly nudge them into moving without thinking about it. They grow gardens and don't have mechanical conveniences for house and yard work."

There are many benefits of regular exercise. Exercise helps you feel better and have more energy. It tones your muscles and tissues for more effective use of strength and nutrients. Exercise increases circulation and delivers oxygen to the cells (remember that cancer doesn't like oxygen). It increases lymphatic flow, which aids in the removal of toxins. It gives you lean muscle mass, improves mental alertness, muscle strength, and stamina. Exercise even helps with digestion of food and assimilation of nutrients. It boosts calorie expenditure and can help with weight loss. Exercise can help you enjoy better sleep, experience greater endurance, have a higher self-esteem, lower cholesterol, build stronger bones, experience less depression, and have a more positive attitude. With all those benefits, why would you put off incorporating exercise into your daily life? Try it, you will like it. And the best exercise is... the one you will do. Just get out and move every day doing something you enjoy. Get a dog to remind you to take walks every day if you need help with this component to health.

I do lead an active lifestyle, but getting consistent exercise was the final health frontier I conquered. I realized about seven years ago that the only way I could make sure I exercised consistently was to get up in the morning and immediately get myself out the door. I found that if I put it off until later in the day, something would always come up and I'd be going to bed at night without having exercised. I had every intention of doing it, but life would get in the way. Doing it first thing in the morning gives you such a satisfaction and gets your day going in the right direction. Fortunately, I have a dog that reminds me every morning to put my shoes on and get going. During the summer months in Florida, we started biking instead of walking because of the heat (I do this in addition to taking the dog for a short walk—she's fifteen). At least with biking you have the wind hitting you and cooling you off a bit. I love our 5-plus-mile bike rides or walks each morning and feel so accomplished after I get home and shower. It's like a load is off my shoulders. I encourage you to make exercise happen first thing in the morning as well, so you won't put it off. Your body and mind will thank you!

I believe the cartoon I licensed from Randy Glasbergen above exemplifies perfectly how important exercise is for human health!

STORY TIME: PATSY BURFORD

"Thank you, Dr. Deb, for this book encouraging us to adopt healthy lifestyle factors such as faith, exercise, hydration, plant-based nutrition, positive thinking, etc. After applying these principles in my own life, I'm now experiencing ultimate health and normal weight at seventy-years-young. I encourage all readers to implement the principles in this book. They make plant-based eating fun, easy, delicious, and exciting!"

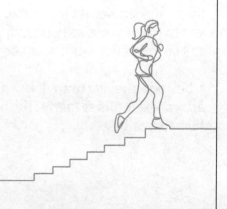

EXERCISE ACTION PLAN

1. Pick five days each week and do some form of exercise first thing in the morning. You can walk, take a bike ride, play tennis with a friend, do yoga, work out at the gym, or anything that gets you moving. If you haven't exercised in a while, start small. If you can only handle five minutes to begin with, then do five minutes, and each week add five more. Do what you can and add more as you are able. Your goal is at least thirty minutes a day.

2. Purposely add more movement into your daily life. Try things like taking the stairs instead of the elevator, parking further out when you go to the store, setting an alarm and doing ten squats every hour, walking around the house while you are on the phone instead of sitting, doing some sit-ups or push-ups while you are watching TV, or doing some deep breathing exercises several times each day.

3. Exercise with a buddy. I was so happy when my husband decided to join me each morning several years ago. I enjoy riding our bikes together and chatting along the way. It is a pleasant way to start the day right for both of us. A buddy can help hold you accountable. One of my bonus (step) daughters, walks and talks to her mom on the phone on her walk. They live in different states but plan their walks together each day. It's a good time for them to connect and hold each other accountable.

4. Buy some kind of exercise tracker to track your activity such as a Fitbit, Garmin or Apple watch. Aim for 10,000 steps per day, starting smaller if you need to.

5. Have fun! Exercise can be quite fun when you get into it, especially when you start seeing some of those benefits I mentioned.

6. As Nike© says, JUST DO IT!

DAILY SUPPORT ACTIONS

Now that you have your health goal established, let's talk about how you can help support yourself to make this goal a reality! It's important to incorporate daily support actions into your goal-setting process to ensure your success. Here are a few that my clients and I have found helpful.

- **Affirmations:** Merriam-Webster Dictionary defines affirmation as "a positive assertion."[126] I already demonstrated how important your thoughts and words are to your happiness and success in life. Positive affirmations can be an important support action to help you achieve your goal, as they program or re-program your subconscious mind. Affirmations engage the mind and emotions. They invite a vibrational energy match that attracts the results to you. Affirmations inspire and motivate you. For affirmations to be effective they need to be:

- **Present tense**: Your subconscious only knows present tense, therefore, state your affirmation as if your goal is already accomplished.

- **Positive**: State the affirmation in the positive instead of negative tense.

- **Short**: Make your statements short and to the point.

- **Specific**: Always be specific so your subconscious doesn't fill in the blank.

---

[126] https://www.merriam-webster.com/dictionary/affirmation

- **Emotional**: Tap into your emotions regarding your goal. Speak the affirmation with emotion.

In the SMART goal example we previously looked at, an effective affirmation would be:

I feel absolutely amazing at _____ pounds (your ideal weight after you lose the desired pounds). I am full of energy and vitality and feel so good about the example I am setting for my family!

- **Prayer:** Prayer is a powerful weapon for all areas of life. Asking for God's help with your goal helps it become a reality. Do you lack discipline? Ask God to help you have discipline. Remember that self-control is a fruit of the spirit. God wants you to be successful and will help if you ask. Of course, it requires your participation. Each moment you feel weak and want to eat something that will not support your goal, ask God for help.

- **Meditation:** No good book on health today would be complete without the topic of meditation. While meditation has been around for thousands of years, we're just starting to understand what is right under our noses, literally! When you learn to focus attention on an object (for example your breath in and out of your lungs), something very interesting starts to happen inside your brain and body. Science is beginning to explain how meditation can help with stress reduction, blood pressure regulation, lowering of cortisol levels, and even pain management. We may never know exactly everything about our brain and how our consciousness works, but what we do know is that meditation works for the brain like exercise does for the body. The more you do, the stronger you become. Rather than build muscle as with exercise, you build attention skills with mediation. These skills allow you to concentrate longer and deeper, have greater depth of clarity, and have better emotional balance, especially during times of stress. Research shows that as these skills improve over time, a sense of happiness independent of conditions begins to emerge and become the default condition. No, this doesn't mean that all your problems go away. It does mean that you become better equipped to deal with the problems. Another metaphor I like to use is that meditation is to daily life what scales are to playing music. Practicing your scales may not be the most fun or glamorous way to spend your time, but when it's time to perform, you'll be happier if you put in the time. My husband, Tim Harrell, is a Level 2 Coach with Unified Mindfulness. He often starts his meditation classes with the short video titled "Wim Hof Method | 'Brain over Body' Michigan Study".[127] The video highlights researchers at Wayne State University showing how meditation can help change physiology. It's been proven that ten minutes of meditation per day on a regular basis is enough to learn one or more techniques and establish a habit. Over time, meditation helps to rewire the brain for better health, success, and happiness. There are many mediation apps to help calm your brain and train it to work for you. A few I like are Headspace, Abide (Christian-based), Calm, and Muse. In a world of ever-increasing distractions, it is important to calm the brain and breathe—really take deep breaths to improve your oxygen. A simple breathing technique is the 5-5-7 breath, where you breathe in through your nose for a count of five seconds, hold the breath in for a count of five seconds, and exhale slowly through your mouth for a count of seven seconds. Repeat ten times per session. When you feel out of control and want to eat to make yourself feel better, try a short meditation or breathing exercise

---

[127] https://www.youtube.com/watch?v=YficBlvPwWQ

instead. Please check out www.contemplatist.com for more info or to get help.

- **Journaling:** A great way to support your health and goals is to journal daily. The benefits of journaling are numerous. Journaling boosts your creativity. Putting pen to paper and writing several pages without stopping can get you in a creative space. I encourage writing whatever comes to mind and not putting much thought into "what" to write. I find it interesting to see what comes up when I do this technique. Ideas often bubble to the surface you weren't aware were there. Journaling helps your emotional health as you work things out on paper. Emptying out your feelings via journaling can help you feel better about what you are dealing with. You can boost your memory by journaling as well. As you write, your brain commits what you are writing to memory. Journaling can be a way of emotionally connecting to your goal. Write about what life will be like when your goal is accomplished. It helps you connect emotionally with your goal, which makes you more likely to accomplish the goal. Some people prefer journaling on a tablet or phone. There are apps you can get to do that. I personally prefer the tactile feel of pen and paper. It's a good exercise to look back on your journals through the years as a reminder of how far you've come. Start journaling today and see the results!

- **Reading and listening to positive books, talks, etc.:** Focusing on positive things will help you stick with your goals by motivating you. It's important to stay in a positive mind frame to accomplish goals. Focusing on the negative in our world is stressful and can contribute to unhealthy habits.

- **Art therapy:** I discovered art therapy in 2011 after my mom passed away. I had always wanted to paint but felt I had practically zero natural talent. When the businesses started popping up where you paint and socialize, I got some friends and went to one of the classes eager to unleash my stuffed creativity. I loved it and even persuaded my husband to go on a date night there. My husband bought me painting classes for my birthday. I went for three hours weekly, and it proved to be incredible therapy for my grief. For three hours a week, I literally got lost in the painting process and didn't think about anything else, especially my sadness. It was incredible, and I highly recommend art therapy to help you live healthier and happier. Many like me feel they don't have talent, but let me assure you, we are all endowed with creativity from our Creator! There is something innate in us to create. You may choose knitting over painting or another form of art and creativity such as music. Just choose something to tap into the creative side of you and reap the amazing benefits!

- **Protecting your environment:** It is important to surround yourself with positive influences, which may require you to limit time with people who don't support your goals. For example, if you have an issue with consuming too much alcohol and want to give it up, you will most likely need to stop hanging around people who like to party. Find people who share your values and goals. It is said that you are the average of the five people closest to you. That is probably true of the average weight, the average motivation, the average morality, etc. If you want to change something in your life, you may need to change other things that contribute to a particular habit, including people and environment. Be willing to set healthy boundaries. You are worth it!

There are other components to health besides nutrition that are just as important and often overlooked. The thoughts you think, the words you speak, how connected you are to your purpose, and whether you have written goals all impact your life and health. Most people coast through life aimlessly not willing to step out of their comfort zone, just to arrive at death's door safely. I encourage you to do whatever work is necessary to discover and tap into your personal purpose. From that I encourage you to set SMART goals in each area of your life. Do the work to transform your toxic thoughts into God-inspired thoughts. Find faith that frees you to be who God has called you to be. Understand that you are loved unconditionally and passionately by the Creator of the universe. Step out in faith knowing God has a bright future for you!

"I have been impressed with the urgency of doing. Knowing is not enough; we must apply. Being willing is not enough; we must do."

Leonardo da Vinci

CHAPTER 6

THRIVAL RESOURCE GUIDE

"Thrive: To grow vigorously: flourish; to progress toward or realize a goal despite or because of circumstances"

Webster's Dictionary[128]

I OFTEN TAKE for granted how easy it is for me to walk out this lifestyle, because I've been at it for so long. I tend to forget that most people have no clue where to start, where to shop, how to substitute ingredients, etc. It is my pleasure to help you navigate implementing this lifestyle, using the knowledge I've gleaned over my many years of plant-based living. This chapter will give you the tools needed to thrive in your journey towards a healthier you. You've learned the why in previous chapters, now I am equipping you with the how.

STOCKING A HEALTHY PANTRY

One thing people often ask me is what I have in my pantry. Here is a partial list of my pantry staples:

---

[128]   https://www.merriam-webster.com/dictionary/thrive

- **Monk fruit sweetener** for baking (mentioned above in the section on sweeteners)

- **Thickener** – I prefer using **arrowroot powder** instead of cornstarch because it is a whole food and relatively unprocessed. It comes from the West Indian arrowroot plant. One tablespoon of arrowroot powder thickens a cup of liquid. It is best to dissolve the powder by stirring it into an equal amount of liquid before adding it to the dish.

- **Baking powder** – Make sure and get the non-aluminum ones, as aluminum is toxic to the brain. Rumford is the brand I use. You can make your own by combining two parts of cream of tartar, one part baking soda (sodium bicarbonate), and two parts arrowroot.

- **Flours** – I recommend avoiding white flour and white flour products. Instead, use whole wheat flour, whole wheat pastry flour, millet flour, buckwheat flour, oat flour, brown rice flour, cassava flour, and gluten-free baking mixes. Semolina flour in pasta is refined, so you want to avoid that as much as possible. Brown rice pastas are my favorite and good for people who are gluten sensitive. My preferred brand is Jovial.

- **Organic cacao powder**–All chocolate products come from the cacao plant, which is an evergreen that grows in Central and South America. Both cacao and cocoa come from the same plant, but they are different. Cocoa, which is common in the US, comes from applying high heat to raw cacao. The heat destroys some vital nutrients this plant contains. For that reason, I prefer using cacao powder instead of cocoa powder in recipes. However, both contain wonderful benefits, so eat up. Cacao (and cocoa to a lesser extent) is a superfood and is an excellent source of calcium, magnesium, fiber, iron, and a plethora of antioxidants. Enjoy it in baking, hot beverages, smoothies, and power balls (see recipes).

- **Dried fruit** – I prefer unsulfured organic ones. Dried fruits are a nice snack when you are craving something sweet. They are also good in baked items, stuffing, and trail mixes. I typically have on hand dried mango, dried figs, Goji berries, raisins, and dates. Remember that if you want or need to lose weight, avoid dried fruits as they are high in calories and natural sugars.

- **Quinoa–**A flowering plant in the amaranth family, quinoa is a staple in South America, especially Peru, where it is grown. I use it instead of rice in dishes. Quinoa is high in protein, dietary fiber, B vitamins, and minerals. It a super food and is lower in starch than rice.

- **Brown rice–**I keep organic brown rice on hand. It is a staple in our family. Make sure and get your rice from California as rice grown in the southern states of the US is high in arsenic, due to the pesticides used on cotton crops nearby. White rice has less arsenic, as most of the arsenic is in the bran, or outer part. I know many people prefer the taste of white rice, but brown rice is more nutritious. I recently started purchasing my organic brown rice from Chico Farms in California. You can find out more at www.chicorice.com.

- **Nutritional yeast** – This is a food supplement high in B vitamins that has a cheesy flavor. It is great sprinkled on popcorn, in soups, sauces, and main dishes. You can find it in the bulk section of the health food store or at places like Vitacost.com. You will see it listed in several of my recipes.

- **Beans–**I always have lots of dried beans of various types on hand including black, pinto, kidney, garbanzo, and lentils, as well as plenty of canned beans. I like the Jovial brand of canned beans because they are in glass jars. The Eden brand is good as well because the lining in their cans is non-toxic. I typically have plenty of those on hand for a quick meal or to throw on salads. Beans are super foods and should be eaten daily. They are overwhelmingly a part of blue zone diets.

- **Popcorn**–Popcorn is a great snack full of fiber. I keep the actual kernels on hand to pop in an air popper or the good old-fashioned way in a pan with a small amount of oil.

- **Salsa**–It's great to have some organic salsa on hand to eat on top of your beans and rice or baked potatoes. Try it, you may like it!

- **Lily's Stevia-Sweetened Chocolate Chips**–I admit, I really like chocolate. It's superb for you too when you eat it without the massive amount of sugar in most chocolates. I keep these chocolate chips on hand for throwing into some banana cookies or to enjoy a handful as a treat.

- **Whole grain pasta**–My favorite pasta is the Jovial brand of brown rice pasta. Pasta is a must in my house as it's my granddaughter's favorite food. It's also great for a quick meal.

- **Marinara sauce**–This is also a must to throw on the above-mentioned pasta or onto a homemade pizza (see recipe). Marinara sauce is also yummy on brown rice or topped on baked potatoes. For a quick soup, I combine a jar of marinara sauce and a can of coconut milk. It makes a yummy and quick cream of tomato soup!

- **Gluten-free tamari sauce** – Tamari is soy sauce made without the wheat. Tamari is typically Japanese and is made from miso (fermented soy paste). To me it seems more robust than soy sauce, which is why I prefer it. I keep it on hand to use in sauces or stir-fries.

- **Herbs and spices** – I keep lots of herbs and spices on hand for cooking. It's a great idea to have a well-rounded supply of these to flavor your food.

- **Spray oil** – I typically don't use oil for cooking but I do like to start sautéing with a spray of oil. I prefer avocado spray oil but any non-hydrogenated, non-GMO one will do.

- **Organic vegetable broth** – This is a must for any kitchen! I use it for sautéing, soups, sauces, and more. I get mine at Costco.

- **Organic applesauce** – I like to have this on hand as I often substitute it for oil in baking recipes.

- **Chia and flaxseeds** – These are great to use in baking, smoothies, or puddings. I aim to eat a tablespoon of one of these each day. Flaxseeds and chia seeds need to be ground before eating as your body won't break them down. Grinding them helps you obtain maximum nutrients from these powerful seeds. I keep a little inexpensive coffee grinder on hand for grinding them. Both are full of plant omega-3 fats and so good for the body and brain! Make sure you eat a tablespoon every day!

KITCHEN NECESSITIES

1. **A good blender** – Vitamix or similar high-powered one.

2. **Instant Pot**—There are other brands too that I'm sure are fine. I use my Instant Pot daily to make rice, beans, soups, etc. An Instant Pot will make your life easier.

3. **A good food processor**—You need this to make hummus, shred veggies, etc.

4. **A glass or stainless-steel electric teapot**—So great for heating water quickly. I recommend one that has adjustable temperature settings as each tea brews best at a certain temperature. I admit, I'm a tea snob!

5. **A waffle iron**—I make my own gluten-free waffles (see recipe) and so this is a must for me. My waffles are not sweet, so I often use them in place of bread. If you want to lose weight, substituting these waffles for bread can help.

6. **Air fryer**—A great way to make "fried" foods without the oil. It's amazing how well it works. I have an air fryer/toaster oven/convection oven combo that I love!

VEGAN EGG SUBSTITUTIONS

Here are a few options to substitute **one egg** in baking:

- Mix 1 tablespoon of ground chia seeds + 3 tablespoons of water. Allow to sit for 5 minutes.

- Mix 1 tablespoon of ground flaxseeds + 3 tablespoons of water. Allow to sit for 5 minutes.

- 1/4 cup of mashed banana

- 1/4 cup of applesauce

- 1/2 mashed avocado

Note: Your choice of which substitute to use will depend on what you are cooking. If you are cooking sweet things like cookies or cakes, then using mashed banana or applesauce will be an excellent choice. If you are baking something savory like cornbread, you will want to use one of the other three options to avoid the sweet flavor.

If you love omelets and quiches and want to enjoy a cruelty-free and cholesterol-free version, try either the Follow Your Heart© or the Just© brands of egg replacers. You can use any of these four in baking:

- Follow Your Heart VeganEgg – www.followyourheart.com
- Just Egg – https://www.ju.st/
- Ener-G Egg Replacer – www.ener-g.com
- Bob's Red Mill Egg Replacer – www.bobsredmill.com

SHOPPING GUIDE

Here is my list of the most affordable places to get some necessities! You can save money living a whole-food plant-based lifestyle!

Organic Produce

1. **Grow your own!** This is the best way to get the freshest organic produce. I have found it to be the best way to get kids to eat more veggies. They love helping to grow and pick the produce. Being involved in the process makes them more likely to eat the fruits and vegetables. You can grow in dirt, in containers on a balcony or patio, or even windowsill. I have found the easiest way to grow produce twelve months out of the year is with an aeroponic vertical growing system called a Tower Garden. We have four Tower Gardens and grow nearly 100% of our greens and herbs and many other

items on them. You can learn more about them at www.
TowerofEden.com. We also grow a bunch of stuff in the
dirt in our small backyard. There's nothing more delicious and nutritious than eating your produce within
minutes of picking!

2. **Farmer's markets or organic co-ops.** This is the sec-
ond-best place to get your organic produce. When you
visit a farmer's market, ask the farmer if the produce
is from their farm or purchased. Sometimes you find
people at farmer's markets who bought produce from
somewhere else to sell. Try and purchase from the
actual farmer if you can. Visiting a farmer's market is a
great experience for the entire family! Co-ops are also
great for getting fresh organic produce. You can typically find them in most cities.

3. **Trader Joe's or Aldi's** can be affordable places to find
organic produce. I prefer Trader Joe's but many people
I know love Aldi's. Be prepared to use the produce
quickly so it does not spoil. You can also find other
deals there!

4. **Costco** is my go-to for things like bananas, avocados,
carrots, berries, squash, zucchini, mushrooms, green
beans, spinach, and asparagus. Each Costco is different,
so you will have to check yours. If you don't grow
your own greens like I do, Costco is typically an excellent source. I also buy all my frozen organic fruits for
smoothies at Costco such as mangos, cherries, strawberries, blueberries, mixed berries, and whatever else
that I find organic there. You absolutely cannot beat
their prices for these things. I also find frozen organic
veggies there such as broccoli, mixed veggies, cauliflower rice, and more. Having these frozen items on
hand is great for quick meals and soups!

5. Sprouts, Natural Grocers, and other health food stores can be good places for many things, especially when they are on sale or BOGO (buy one get one free). I've found Sprouts to have decent prices on organic produce most of the year. Of course, it depends on what you have available in your area. Publix, Kroger, HEB, and other stores are providing a lot of plant-based options now as well. You can download their apps and watch for what's on sale.

Other Items – Costco

As I mentioned in the above section, every Costco is different so check your local store. These are the items I typically buy at Costco:

- Dave's Killer Bread
- Organic pasta
- Organic marinara
- Organic peanut and almond butters
- Walnuts, almonds, organic chia, hemp and pumpkin seeds
- Seaweed snacks
- Organic salsa
- Organic hummus
- Himalayan salt
- Organic spices
- Organic dried beans

- Canned natural black olives
- Kalamata olives and hearts of palm
- Dr. Praeger's veggie burgers
- Beyond Burgers
- Organic quinoa
- Organic canned beans
- Non-toxic laundry detergent
- Organic soy and oat milks

Vitacost – an Online Health Food Store

I order non-perishables monthly on www.Vitacost.com as their prices can't be beat. They offer free shipping on orders of at least $49. I typically receive my shipment within a few days, which is nice! It's convenient, fast, and affordable. Prices will typically be lower than local health food stores. I love to support local and do that with perishable items. With non-perishables, you can't beat Vitacost.

Other Places to Shop

Here are a few other places I shop for various items:

- **www.JovialFoods.com**–I buy organic Einkorn flour, brown rice pasta (they have the best), glass-jarred tomatoes (it's better to not get these in cans because tomatoes are so acidic), and glass-jarred beans. Please note that I always choose glass jars over cans when possible. Cans often contain BPA (bisphenol A), BPS (bisphenol S), BPF (bisphenol F), or phthalate in their linings. These are industrial chemicals and studies have shown they are toxic to our bodies. They appear in plastic containers, personal care products, and cash register receipts. If you'd like to read more about what the studies have shown, go to www.EWG.org or visit this article (https://www.healthline.com/nutrition/what-is-bpa#exposure) which sites several studies. Also, please note that several countries have banned these products which speaks volumes. One of the best brands to buy in cans is Eden Foods. They have been a frontrunner in getting rid of toxic chemicals from their products since 1999.

- **www.ChicoRice.com**–As I mentioned earlier, this is where I have found the freshest organic brown rice. A 20-pound bag is $42, and that includes shipping. The rice is grown on a family-owned farm in California. So yummy!

- **www.Crunchi.com/healthpeak**–A big source of toxins in our world comes from personal care products. Typically, women are exposed to more toxic chemicals than men because there are many harmful chemicals in make-up. Over the years, I have tried many "natural" skin care and makeup lines, often walking away disappointed. It seemed the cleaner the line, the less they worked like I wanted. And then there is the whole green-washing issue—companies acting like they are "clean and green" but not really being all that clean and green when you analyze the ingredients. The other issue I found was that many lines still test on animals, which is against my conviction—or they are not vegan, again against my conviction. I was so excited when I found Crunchi, a line of truly clean and green personal care and cosmetic products that are not only good for your body but are outstanding quality that keeps you looking good all day. The company is women-founded and operated and has a noble mission. I am proud to recommend Crunchi to my friends, family and clients. They make Crunchi products with a combination of safe, certified-organic, and EcoCert ingredients. Using years of compiled, evidence-based research and safety data, Crunchi has thoughtfully selected ingredients that will not put your health at risk. To check to see if the products you are using are truly safe, go to www.EWG.org and check. You no longer need to compromise your health for your beauty, or your beauty for your health with Crunchi!

THE CASE FOR SUPPLEMENTS

In a perfect world, with perfect nutrition, a pure environment, zero stress, and daily exercise, supplements would not be necessary. We do not live in a perfect world. Our food, habits and environment, including electromagnetic fields and other forms of radiation and toxins, limit our body's natural ability to maintain peak health. As a result, many of us, including children, can benefit from various supplements and therapies designed to help bring us back into balance.

Although I normally tailor supplements to people based on many factors, there are several mainstays I believe most of us need. They are as follows:

- **Digestive enzymes**–Take only when eating cooked food. Raw food has enzymes, so when eating raw food, taking enzymes is unnecessary. Digestive enzymes turn the food we eat into energy used for various biological processes. Cooking destroys the enzymes in the food, so when you eat cooked food, it's beneficial to take digestive enzymes.

- **Apple Cider Vinegar (ACV)**–Organic, raw and with the "mother" (I prefer the Bragg's brand). The "mother" of apple cider vinegar is the culture of beneficial bacteria that turns regular apple cider into vinegar in the first place (it will look like sediment at the bottom of the bottle). Take 1 tablespoon every morning in a big glass of water. Follow that with a little water to rinse your mouth to protect your tooth enamel. If you would like to lose weight, incorporate 2 teaspoons of vinegar into every meal according to Michael Greger, MD, in his book *How Not to Diet* (which I highly recommend). He says to use any vinegar for the weight loss, but ACV is the most nutritious of any vinegar, so that's what I recommend for optimal health. Here are some benefits of ACV:

  - Helps to prevent mouth canker sores
  - Promotes a healthy pH balance in the body
  - Helps control weight
  - Removes toxins
  - Anti-aging
  - Maintains healthy skin (use 1-part ACV + 1-part purified water for an excellent skin toner)
  - Helps with heartburn and other digestive disorders

- **Vitamin D3/K2**–When we are young, we can convert sunshine into Vitamin D in the body. As we age, we can't do that conversion very well and it becomes necessary to supplement. Kids can often benefit from Vitamin D supplementation if they don't spend consistent time in sunshine every day. Vitamin D improves the immune system, helps reduce the risk of cardiovascular disease, and strengthens bones and muscles. Vitamin D3 is the best form to take and combining it with Vitamin K2 works with D to keep calcium out of the blood and in the bones. There are many medical opinions about ideal Vitamin D blood levels. The recommendations vary from 20 ng/ml to between 40 and 60 ng/ml. Most people can get by with taking 2000 IU per day of Vitamin D3 but may need to up the amount as they age and during winter months. Of course, children take less, depending on their age.

- **Whole-food based vitamin/mineral supplements**–If you juice a variety of vegetables every day, you should not need one of these. If you have a perfect diet and digestive system, you should not need these. If you don't do those two things, you probably need a whole-food concentrate to supplement what is missing in your diet. Here are the options I suggest: 1) **Juice Plus+** concentrated fruits and vegetables in capsules or gummies which has a wonderful program where kids, including college kids, can get free product for up to four years. It's a great deal and something I have been recommending since 2002. You can learn more about it at drdeb.juiceplus.com or talk to someone you know who uses it. 2) **Barley Green**–powdered barley grass has many health benefits. Many people don't like the taste of Barley Green and therefore might consider one of the other options. I like it mixed in a little water. 3) Optimal Health Systems has a whole food based Vitamin/Mineral supplement I recommend. Contact me if you are interested in this one. 4) Dr. Fuhrman has good quality food-based supplements for men and women. You can find those at www.drfuhrman.com.

- **Zinc**–Many people are deficient in zinc. Zinc helps your immune system and helps prevent the flu, coronavirus, etc. I recommend 30-50 milligrams per day of organic zinc.

- **Turmeric**–A root that is a great spice used in Indian cooking that has many health benefits. Turmeric is a great anti-inflammatory, is excellent for the brain, and helps kill viruses. Curcumin, which gives turmeric its bold yellow color, is the real powerhouse in turmeric. Several studies have been done on curcumin, and there is promising data showing it can help prevent and even arrest cancer growth, and a host of other things. Take 1/4 to 1 teaspoon of turmeric powder daily, depending on your situation. The nutrients are fat soluble and 300 times more potent when combined with black pepper, so I recommend mixing it in a little almond or peanut butter and a bit of honey or maple syrup after a meal when you have had a little black pepper. You can also just add the black pepper to the mixture. You don't need a lot of black pepper, just a couple sprinkles or grinds from a pepper grinder. Plus, it makes an OK little dessert! You may need more depending on your issue (such as arthritis) and may want to choose a supplement.

- **Homeopathic Remedies**–I got introduced to homeopathy when my daughter Cristina was in first grade, as I mentioned in my introduction. I am a firm believer in the power of homeopathy to help boost your body to do its job. The book I recommend every home have is *Everybody's Guide to Homeopathic Medicines* by Stephen Cummings, MD, and Dana Ullman, MPH. You may want to consider purchasing some basic homeopathy kits to have on hand. If you have children, the children's homeopathy kit is a must.

If you'd like to explore other supplements to help your body heal, you can set up a virtual consultation with me to develop your personal plan. You can reach me at www.PureLightHealth.com.

DETOXIFY YOUR HOME

Another reason women's exposure to toxins is greater than men's is because they are usually the ones who do most of the housecleaning. Mostly, but of course, many men help with household chores. There are many toxins lurking in most household cleaners. Exposure happens by breathing them as you clean, and through your skin if you don't use gloves. We know many of the chemicals in these cleaners to be carcinogenic.

Another source of toxins in and around the home comes in the form of pesticides used to control bugs in the home and yard. Don't think that monthly pest service you pay decent money for does not come without challenges. There are several studies showing increased cancer risk in both children and adults exposed to these pesticides. You can find a great article highlighting these studies at: https://www.cancertherapyadvisor.com/home/tools/fact-sheets/pesticides-and-cancer/ I will not go into them here, but will provide alternatives for you to consider. In most cities you can find companies that provide non-toxic pest care. They often use things like diatomaceous earth (DE) and boric acid. Both are very effective against bugs. They typically only must treat your home once per year and guarantee results.

I highly recommend you get rid of all toxins. Remember, there are two causes of disease: nutritional deficiencies and toxicity. Personal care products, cleaning products, food, and pesticides in the home can all be causes of toxicity in your body. Obviously, we can't avoid all toxins, no matter how diligent we are, but we can control what we can control.

HOME CLEANING PRODUCTS AND RECIPES

All-Purpose Cleaner:

- 2 teaspoons aluminum-free baking soda + 1/2 teaspoon non-toxic dish soap (such as Ecos or Seventh Generation) + 4 tablespoons white vinegar + several drops of lemon, tea tree, eucalyptus, or lavender essential oils.

- I use the EnviroCloth and the window micro-fiber cloths from Norwex. You can purchase them from my friend Patsy at https://patsyburford.norwex.biz. You can pretty much clean everything with these two cloths. Norwex's claim to fame is that they remove 99% of bacteria from the surface with just water. You can read about their technology on the website. I'm a big fan of these and have two sets placed in different locations in my home.

Glass Cleaner:

- 2 cups of water + 1/4 cup of white vinegar mixed in a spray bottle.

- Instead of any cleaner, the Norwex cloths mentioned above will clean windows and glass (with just water) better than anything I've ever seen.

Dusting Spray:

- 2 teaspoons of olive oil + 1 teaspoon lemon or orange essential oil + 1/4 cup white vinegar + 1 cup warm water.

- I dust with the Norwex dusting mitt instead. It's much easier and furniture looks great after!

Carpet Cleaner:

- 1 tablespoon of Borax + 1 small box of aluminum-free baking soda. Mix and sprinkle on the rug and then vacuum.

Floor Cleaner:

- 1/4 cup white vinegar + 1 tablespoon non-toxic dish soap + 1/4 cup aluminum-free baking soda + 2 gallons of water.

- I use the Norwex mop and water instead.

Toilet Cleaner:

- 2 cups water + 1/4 cup liquid Castile soap + 4 drops lavender essential oil + 4 drops tea tree oil + 4 drops lemon oil. Mix in a spray bottle and spray the toilet. Let sit for 30 minutes and scrub, brush and flush!

Dust Mites:

- Mix 2 cups water + 2 cups white vinegar + 15 drops eucalyptus essential oil. Spray onto pillows and mattresses. Let air dry.

Room Spray:

- Glass spray bottle + water + witch hazel (use 1/5 the amount of water you use) + essential oil of choice (number of drops depends on size of bottle you use— if you use a 2-ounce size bottle, then you will use 10-15 drops of essential oil). This works great as an air freshener in the bathroom. Febreze, Glade, and those other sprays are toxic! You also can get some already made natural sprays such as Citrus Magic, but it is easy and inexpensive to make your own.

- Room essential oil diffuser—water + essential oils of choice.

- You can simmer a pan of water on top of the stove with a chopped-up orange (peel included), cinnamon sticks, and cloves. Keep adding water for several days to the same mix. Refresh every few days. It's delightful, especially at the holidays!

EATING OUT AND SOCIAL SITUATIONS

Eating out as a plant-based person is so much easier now than when I started this journey in 1976. Back then it was almost impossible to eat out, at least eat something good out! Often it was a salad and a plain baked potato. Now most restaurants have vegan options and if you don't see them on the menu, just ask and the chef is often happy to oblige. They estimate that nearly ten million Americans are now vegan, up three hundred percent in the past fifteen years. This is about three percent of the population. The movement is reaching the tipping point, as evidenced by how many plant-based options occupy grocery store shelves and restaurant menus.

Obviously, there are areas in the country where the options for plant-based foods are better than others. For example, in rural Alabama the options are slim, while in large cities (most of them anyway), options abound!

Even when you attend conferences and meetings, you can request a vegan meal. I have been active in helping raise awareness in organizations for the need for offering good options for plant-based people. I have left events where the meat-eaters got this abundant gourmet meal, and the vegans got a salad and a few pieces of asparagus and a little bit of potatoes. I left frustrated and hungry. Hence, I got involved with the organizers and let them know politely that just because we are vegan does not mean we don't like to have a substantial meal. Don't feel bad asking for what you need.

When you get invited to people's houses for dinner, don't be bashful about informing them of your dietary restrictions. You can let them know that for health reasons you are eating a plant-based diet. It is true, eating this way is for your health. If you had celiac disease, you would not hesitate to let them know you can't eat any gluten. People have no problem adjusting the meal to accommodate you. I tell people that a salad and baked potato are some of my favorite things, and it would delight me to have just that. Getting together with other people really is not so much about what food you eat, but about the fellowship anyway. I always ask people when I invite them to dinner if they have any allergies, dietary restrictions, or foods they don't like. I want to make something my guests can enjoy, so I make sure and check with them before I decide on the menu. I suppose I'm more sensitive to this because I have lived this lifestyle for so long! I promise you; you will not offend people if you let them know your dietary restrictions. And who knows, your example may influence them to adopt a healthier plant-strong lifestyle.

I recommend the **Happy Cow** app for your phone which helps to find vegetarian and vegan-friendly restaurants wherever you go. It's a great resource that makes traveling easy. I've only found a few places along the way where I could find absolutely nothing I could eat on the menu. Typically, barbecue places have nothing, but I just avoid those places. I don't have an issue with fasting a meal if I can't find anything. Eating out or with other people is very doable in our world today. The only requirement is being willing to ask for what you want. Most businesses want to please their customers and are more than willing to accommodate you.

EAT AN ALKALINE DIET

As I mentioned earlier, the ideal diet is eighty percent alkaline and only twenty percent acidic. Here is a chart showing which foods fall into each category to help you.

Acid Ash Foods	Alkaline Ash Foods
Some Raw Fruits and Vegetables (cranberries, blueberries, plums, prunes, squash)	Raw Fruits
Whole Grains - Cooked	Dried Fruits
Overcooked Fruits and Vegetables	Raw Vegetables
Dairy Products (Cheese, Milk, Yogurt, Eggs)	Frozen Fruits and Vegetables
Sugar and Refined Grains	Lightly Steamed Fruits and Vegetables
White Meats (fish and foul)	Raw Nuts (almonds, cashews, pecans, walnuts, etc.)
Red Meats (beef, pork, and mutton)	Raw Seeds (sesame, pumpkin, flax, chia, sunflower, etc.)
Herbs, Spices, Condiments, Spicy Foods (onions, garlic, hot peppers, horseradish, etc.)	Sprouted Grains
Fried Foods	
Coffee and Tea	
Alcohol (beer, wine, etc.)	
Drugs and Medications	
Tobacco	

MY RECOMMENDED HEALTH VIDEOS

Title	Source/Author	Where to Watch
Forks Over Knives	https://www.forksoverknives.com/the-film/	Can rent on Amazon Prime, iTunes, YouTube
How Not to Die	Michael Greger, MD	https://youtu.be/7rNY7xKyGCQ
How Not to Diet	Michael Greger, MD	https://nutritionfacts.org/video/evidence-based-weight-loss-live-presentation/
What the Health	https://www.whatthehealthfilm.com	Netflix
The Game Changers	https://gamechangersmovie.com	Netflix
Plant Pure Nation	https://www.plantpurenation.com	https://youtu.be/yBKnG9Y0owQ
Fat, Sick and Nearly Dead	Joe Cross	https://www.rebootwithjoe.com/joes-films/
Cowspiracy - The Sustainability Secret	https://www.cowspiracy.com	Netflix
Food Inc.	http://www.takepart.com/foodinc/index.html	http://www.documentarymania.com/player.php?title=Food%20Inc
Dying to Have Known	www.gerson.org	https://www.youtube.com/watch?v=-FCJGNmmb0oandt=13s

MY RECOMMENDED HEALTH BOOKS

Title	Source/Author	Main Topic
The China Study	T. Colin Campbell, PhD	Cancer
Whole:Rethinking the Science of Nutrition	T. Colin Campbell, PhD	Nutrition science
How Not to Diet	Michael Greger, MD	Evidence-based weight loss
How Not to Die	Michael Greger, MD	How to prevent and reverse the top killers in America
Dr. Neal Barnard's Program for Reversing Diabetes (also cookbook)	Neal Barnard, MD	Diabetes
Power Foods for the Brain	Neal Barnard, MD	Preventing dementia, etc.
Your Body in Balance	Neal Barnard, MD	Hormone health
Prevent and Reverse Heart Disease	Caldwell Esselstyn, MD	Cardiovascular disease
The Starch Solution	John McDougall, MD	Weight loss with starch-based foods
The Plant Based Solution	Joel Kahn, MD	Overall health and wellness
Diet for a New America	John Robbins	Overall health and wellness
The Alzheimer's Solution	Dean and Ayesha Sherzai, MD's	Brain health
Proteinaholic	Garth Davis, MD	How our obsession with meat is killing us and what we can do about it
Eat to Live	Joel Fuhrman, MD	Nutritarian weight loss

MY FAVORITE PERSONAL & SPIRITUAL GROWTH BOOKS

Title	Source/Author	Main Topic
The Greatest Miracle in the World	Og Mandino (my all-time favorite author!)	My #1 recommended book-contains the God Memorandum to you!
Return of the Ragpicker	Og Mandino	Sequel to The Greatest Miracle
Win The Day	Mark Batterson	7 daily habits to help you stress less & accomplish more
Reaching For the Invisible God, What Can We Expect to Find?	Philip Yancey	Deep, satisfying insights to the questions you often are afraid to ask.
The Traveler's Gift	Andy Andrews	7 decisions that determine success
The Shack	Wm. Paul Young	A grieving father confronts God with desperate questions & finds unexpected answers—powerful!
Whisper	Mark Batterson	The 7 ways God speaks to us
The 4:8 Principle	Tommy Newberry	The secret to a joy-filled life
If You Want to Walk on Water You've Got to Get Out of the Boat	John Ortberg	Discover your incredible potential outside your comfort zone
Hinds Feet on High Places	Hannah Hurnard	An allegory of Christian living
How to Win Friends & Influence People	Dale Carnegie	Improves emotional intelligence
Switch on Your Brain	Dr. Caroline Leaf	The key to peak happiness, thinking & health

There are thousands of books I could recommend but these are some of my favorites. Make reading a part of your daily habit.

Remember that "leaders are readers" and "readers are leaders."
I urge you to stay in a constant state of growth. It will enrich
your life in ways you can't imagine.

RECOMMENDED RECIPE AND PLANT-BASED RESOURCES

Website	Source/Author	Resources
www.PCRM.org	Physician's Committee for Responsible Medicine	Excellent downloads available on many topics as well as recipes!
www.PlantPureNation.com	T. Colin Campbell, PhD and family	Meal delivery service, recipes and classes
www.NutritionFacts.org	Michael Greger, MD	Most comprehensive database on nutrition and health! Videos, resources.
www.Benbellavegan.com	BenBella Books	Great recipes
www.FatFreeVegan.com		Fat-free vegan recipes
www.DrMcDougall.com	John McDougall, MD	Health programs and resources He also has an app you can download.
www.ForksOverKnives.com	Forks Over Knives	Excellent recipes and resources
www.TheCulinaryGym.com	Chef Katie Mae (chef for True North and Dr. McDougall)	Classes and recipes
www.thisrawsomeveganlife.com www.rawmazing.com www.FullyRaw.com	Various	Raw recipes and resources
www.Pinterest.com	Pinterest	Follow me! Great resource for recipes. Just type in vegan _____
www.OhSheGlows.com	Angela Liddon	Great recipes and has an app!
www.TCDrCarol.com	Carol Watson, ND, RN, and Body Confidence Coach	Transformational coaching for weight loss and life! I highly recommend!
www.KailoNutrition.com	Heather Borders, RD	Resources and recipes
www.FoodRevolution.org	John and Ocean Robbins	Great recipes and resources
www.TheNeuroPlan.com	Dean and Ayesha Sherzai, MD's	Recipes and resources for brain health
www.PetaLambs.com	Persons for the Ethical Treatment of Animals from a Christian perspective	Resources and info on why you may want to consider veganism as a Christian
www.VeganHealth.org	Plant-based dietitians	Evidence-based nutrient recommendations
www.JewishVeg.org	Rabbis encourage going plant-based	Recipes and resources from a Jewish perspective
www.VeganYogaLife.com	Taylor	Recipes and resources
www.NutriPlanet.org	Nele Liivlaid	Vegan candida guide and recipes
www.Sakara.com	Various MD's	Organic, plant-based meal delivery services and resources
www.PlantBasedDoctors.org	PCRM	A resource to find plant-based doctors in your area!
www.DrFuhrman.com	Joel Fuhrman, MD	Nutritarian Lifestyle

DR. DEB'S TOP TEN HEALTHY HACKS

In today's world, we want shortcuts. We live in a microwave society where people want instant this and that. We want quick answers and quick solutions to whatever issue we are facing. We don't have the understanding that good health is like growing bamboo. You must build the structure, the roots, and the foundation, to grow and flourish. Natural healing is a process that takes time and effort. There really are no short-cuts to anything worth having. And so it is, especially with health. As Jack Lalane said on his 90th birthday, "You have to work at living, because dying is easy." But there are ways to make the process more efficient, effective, and doable in today's fast-paced world. I call these ways healthy hacks. Here are my suggested Healthy Hacks to help make this whole-food plant-pure lifestyle doable for you:

1. **Power Up on Produce** – This is the single most important recommendation I can give you to improve your health, as I have already stated. It is so important that it bears repeating. You want to eat a colorful diet full of micro-nutrients! Remember that there are over 12,000 micronutrients in fruits and vegetables. You want to eat a variety every day from every color, and you need 7-13 servings per day minimal, the more the better.

2. **Be Prepared** – I cannot overstate the importance of being prepared with healthy food, so you avoid grab-bing whatever junk you can get your hands on. When people are hungry, they grab what they can. Therefore, make sure there are plenty of good things to grab. Keep cut up veggies on hand such as carrots, celery, red, yellow and green pepper slices, cucumbers, etc., all in glass jars filled with water (to keep them fresh) or in plastic containers or baggies. You can buy baby carrots and grape tomatoes that are excellent to have on hand. Other items to keep handy are individual hummus

containers, avocado mash (Costco), and homemade dips, and spreads to eat with your raw veggies. Fruit is the best fast food so keep plenty of pieces of fruit around to grab when you want something sweet or individual baggies of grapes, berries, etc. Accessibility is key! Have them available when you need to grab and go or grab and eat. Spend some time on the weekend to prep these snacks to have them available. You can also prep things to cook with during the week like diced onions, garlic and other veggies.

3. **Enjoy a Green Smoothie Daily** – Smoothies are a great way to get a bunch of plants into your diet every day! They can also be an easy way to get kids to eat things like raw spinach or kale. I have some recipes on my website at www.PureLightHealth.com for green smoothies. The basic recipe is eight ounces of water or plant-based milk, one banana, one cup raw spinach or kale, one cup of frozen organic berries, mango, or pineapple, and one tablespoon of chia or ground flaxseeds. If you don't use frozen fruit, then add some ice cubes. Blend well and enjoy. You can add leftover smoothies to popsicle molds for a delicious and healthy popsicle. Experiment with ingredients and have fun exploring the possibilities. If you want it sweeter, add three to four dates. This makes a perfect on-the-go breakfast!

4. **Incorporate Salads in a Jar** – Have you ever heard of a salad-in-a-jar or a salad-in-a-jar party? This is a perfect way to make sure to eat a healthy salad every day! Get some quart mason jars and chop up a bunch of lettuce (or use spring mix or spinach) and veggies that you love in your salad. Make some homemade dressings or buy a healthy dressing such as Bragg's vinaigrette. Set out five jars for Monday through Friday. Place the dressing in the bottom of the jars followed by the hardest veggies such as cut up carrots and celery. Then add softer

veggies such as grape tomatoes. You can also add some beans such as garbanzos, dried cranberries, sunflower or pumpkin seeds, or one-fourth cup of walnuts. Top with the lettuce, spinach, or spring mix. Cap and place in the refrigerator. Each day grab a jar to take to work with you and have it for lunch. Simply shake the jar to disperse the dressing and then dump it in a large bowl and enjoy! Host a salad-in-a-jar party and have everyone bring their own jars and different toppings for everyone to share. It's super fun and encourages others to eat salad daily!

5. **Sip On Soup**–I love soup! Soup is a great way to get a healthy meal all year long. Often, especially in the winter, we have soup and salad for dinner. There are so many healthy, wonderful plant-based soups to enjoy. I have included several recipes for them in Chapter 7. A great way to ensure healthy meals during the week is to make a big pot of soup on the weekend and have it throughout the week, either for lunch or dinner. Soups are a great way to get vegetables, beans, and grains into your diet. Sipping on soup helps you eat slower, which improves digestion and enhances metabolism. Soup is also very filling, so it keeps you from wanting more after mealtime. Make a batch of soup and sip on it throughout the week.

6. **Fill Up on Fiber**–Fiber is the part of fruits, vegetables, beans, and grains that you cannot digest. It acts as an intestinal broom or mop, moving the waste out! Fiber takes the garbage out of your body for you. Trust me, you want the garbage out! Fiber binds dietary cholesterol and moves it out of the body, which as you can imagine is so important for your health. Fiber slows the release of sugar into the blood and prevents hunger and aids in weight loss. As Henry Wheeler Shaw said, "A good reliable set of bowels is worth far more to a

man than any quantity of brains." I cannot overstate the benefits of a fiber-rich diet. Massive scientific evidence concludes fiber helps prevent cancer, especially colorectal cancer, which is the fastest growing cancer in our country. Do you realize your colon is five to six feet long and your small intestines are about twenty-two to twenty-four feet long? Think about how much twisting and turning must happen in the space of your gut for approximately thirty feet of intestines to fit in. Fiber keeps everything moving through all those feet of territory. There are two types of fiber, and we need both for optimal health. Insoluble fiber does not hold water and acts like a broom moving through your gut. It adds bulk to the stool and seems to move food more quickly through the stomach and intestines. We find insoluble fiber in things like wheat bran, vegetables, and whole grains. Soluble fiber holds water and turns to gel during digestion. It acts like a mop moving through your intestines. Soluble fiber comes from chia and flax seeds, psyllium husks, beans, oat bran, nuts, lentils, and some fruits and vegetables. Fiber is filling and will keep you from wanting more than you need. Each meal should have an abundance of fiber, and a whole-food plant-based lifestyle has sufficient fiber. When people ask you where you get your protein on a plant-based diet, ask them where they get their fiber.

7. **Stay Hydrated** – Unfortunately, dehydration is rampant amongst Americans! I really should not have to talk about the importance of water in a healthy lifestyle, but sometimes the simplest of things is the hardest for people to incorporate. Drinking water seems to be one of the difficult things for many of my clients, especially the older ones. I used to deal with this issue with my mom for several years before she passed away. Her legs would often swell, and I told her it was because she was dehydrated. She found this hard to believe, so

I challenged her the next day to drink one-half of her body weight in ounces of water. The way I got her to accomplish that was I measured out the amount she needed to drink in the morning and told her that her goal was to drink it all during the day. She accepted the challenge and commented to me the next day that she had no swelling. It was like magic! The body will hold on to water when it is not getting enough. Once you give it what it needs, it releases the water. It seems counter-intuitive, but I promise you, it is the truth. Headaches are often a result of not drinking enough water. When you get a headache, why do you take an aspirin or ibuprofen? Do you have an aspirin or ibuprofen deficiency? Of course, you don't. Instead of reaching for the drug, try drinking a large glass of water (or several) instead. The result may pleasantly surprise you! As we age our thirst mechanism fades so we can't rely on that in our older years. We must measure out how much water we need—I recommend one-half of your body weight in ounces of water per day, more if you sweat or drink coffee and alcohol. Water does so many important things in the body. Next to oxygen, it is the most important thing that your body needs. You can go without food for many days, but you cannot go without water for very long. Water helps to regulate body temperature, deliver nutrients and oxygen to your cells, remove wastes from cells, cushion your joints, protect your organs and tissues, prevent and relieve constipation, and moistens tissues in the eyes, nose, and mouth. Now that you know all of that, will you stay well-hydrated? I hope so! A great electrolyte drink I learned from Marilyn Joyce, RD, is to take a gallon of pure water and squeeze one lemon, one lime, and one orange into it. It's delicious and helps those people who say they don't like the taste of water. And sorry Gatorade, this is a much better electrolyte drink—all natural, nutritious, and delicious. How do you know if you are drinking enough water? Look at the color of your urine. You want it the color of light straw. The darker it is, the more dehydrated you are. Drink up!

8. **Keep Track—**Whatever you want to change, track. Tracking brings awareness which facilitates change. If you go to a financial person to give you advice on how to manage your money, they are going to encourage you to keep track of what you are spending. As it is with your health. If you want to get healthier and/or lose weight, you need to keep track of what you are eating, how much water you are drinking, etc. Tracking brings awareness and allows you to know where you may falter. You may think you eat a lot of fruits and veggies, but when you track how much, you may find you did not eat as many as you thought you did. That is why I love Dr. Greger's Daily Dozen app. It helps you keep track. I highly recommend you download that free app and start keeping track of your habits!

9. **Get an Accountability Buddy—**One of the best ways to make this journey fun is to find a buddy to do it with. Your buddy should be someone you know who has similar health goals to you. They should be a positive influence on you and someone you enjoy being around. You can hold each other accountable to the healthy habits, share recipes, take walks together (if you live in the same city—or you can talk on the phone while you both walk in your locations), encourage one another, and celebrate your progress. Having someone hold you accountable to the things you say you will do can motivate you to stay on track. Competitive people benefit from participating in a contest with other people. Whatever works for you, do what will help guarantee your success. Having a buddy can help with that!

10. **Keep a Gratitude Journal**– If you have never kept a gratitude journal, then the time is now. The Merriam-Webster Dictionary defines gratitude as "the state of being grateful: thankfulness."[129] I have kept a gratitude journal two separate years in the last ten years, and the practice is truly life-transforming. You can use any journal as a gratitude journal. I kept mine on my nightstand next to my bed, and before I would go to bed at night, I would pull it out and write five things that I was grateful for that day. I tried to think of different things every day that I was grateful for that I had not written before. Doing that for 365 days made me look for the most minute things to be grateful for and write them in my journal that night. For example, I wrote things like: "I'm grateful for hot water in my shower.", "I'm grateful for the sound of the birds chirping.", "I'm grateful that I can hear my granddaughter's laughter.", "I'm grateful I can see that sunset.", "I'm grateful I have the physical capability to take this walk.", "I'm grateful for the flowers blooming.", "I'm grateful for this pain I'm feeling because it helps me know how wonderful it is when I don't have pain." Gratitude is a practice that can literally change your life! I expressed gratitude for the large blessings in my life (my family, etc.) but also for the tiny blessings. When you adopt the habit of perpetual gratitude, it transforms your attitude, countenance, and your life. Get a journal and start today writing five things you are grateful for this day. Do this for a period of a year, then write to me and tell me how it transformed your life. I promise it will, and it will help you have better health too!

---

[129] https://www.merriam-webster.com/dictionary/gratitude

ACTION PLAN

1. Choose two of these tips and incorporate them this week!
2. Make one of the healthy cleaning recipes.
3. Check out three websites from my recommendations.
4. Try two new recipes from this book or one of the sites.
5. Start your gratitude journal!

The resources I have put in this chapter are meant to help you implement my recommendations easily. Tap into the plethora of available information I have listed to educate and inspire you to make the changes to help your body heal. You are meant not just to survive, but to THRIVE! These resources will equip you for thriving. You will be glad you put in the time and effort to make the necessary changes. Thriving is so much better than simply surviving!

CHAPTER 7

DR. DEB'S DELICIOUS RECIPES

Let your food be your medicine and your medicine be your food.

GOD OFTEN SPEAKS to me using examples found in nature. I have a couple of bird feeders in my yard and can sit for hours watching them. We have birds here in Florida called Nuthatches. They are cool little birds, except they can be a menace at a bird feeder as they use their beak to sift through the seeds, looking for the ones they like the most. Consequently, a bunch of the seeds land on the ground, which pleases the squirrels in my yard, but not me.

Looking for a healthy recipe you enjoy can be like a Nuthatch sifting through the seeds in a bird feeder. You look and look, tossing the ones you think you won't like, until you find one that looks appetizing. But sometimes, despite how beautiful the author's pictures look or how wonderful people say the dish is, you spend the time and energy to make something and end up disappointed.

My goal in this chapter is to do the sifting for you. Remember that I've been plant-based since 1976, so I have a ton of experience in the kitchen cooking for my family and friends. I love feeding people healthy vegan fare! We've tested a lot of recipes that didn't satisfy or didn't turn out as they should have. My recipes here have stood the test of time and pleased many guests at my kitchen table over the years. Most are pretty kid and picky-eater friendly. Most are even enjoyed by big meat eaters. I bring these to you confidently knowing that you will enjoy them. The recipes are not only delicious, but nutritious as well. These recipes can provide medicine to your body and satisfaction to your taste buds! Enjoy!

Please note that although I don't say organic for every one of these ingredients, I always recommend organic whenever possible, especially for the items I mentioned in the section on organic.

BREAKFAST RECIPES

Raw Applesauce

For a delicious and nutritious breakfast or snack, try this raw applesauce. You can also use it on top of toast or oatmeal.

Recipe serves: 6

Ingredients:

- 4 organic apples
- 1 tablespoon fresh lemon juice
- Ground cinnamon to taste, optional

Directions:

1. Blend all ingredients together in a blender or food processor.
2. Place in a glass container and chill before serving.

Chocolate Chia Pudding

This pudding is full of nutrients and essential fats. It makes a great breakfast topped with fresh fruit and can be enjoyed as a yummy dessert.

Optional add-ons: Cinnamon, nutmeg, unsweetened coconut, pumpkin or sunflower seeds, hemp hearts, fresh fruit, cacao nibs

Recipe serves: 6

Ingredients:

- 1.5 cups plant-based milk: almond, cashew, oat, etc.
- 1/3 cup chia seeds
- 5-7 Medjool dates
- ¼ cup cacao powder

Directions:

1. Blend all ingredients together in a blender or food processor.
2. Place in a glass container or glass serving bowls and chill before serving.

Energy Balls

These are decadent and can be enjoyed at breakfast with some fresh fruit or as a healthy dessert or snack anytime. Just make sure and not eat too many as they are calorie dense.

Recipe serves: 25

Ingredients:

- 2 cups organic rolled oats
- 4 tablespoons ground chia seeds or flaxseeds
- 1 cup peanut or almond butter
- 6 tablespoons shredded unsweetened coconut
- 4 tablespoons pure maple syrup
- ½ cup organic raisins
- ½ cup vegan chocolate chips

Directions:

1. Combine all ingredients together in a large bowl.
2. Roll into balls and roll in cacao powder or ground flax-seeds for extra nutrition.
3. Store in the refrigerator or freezer (I prefer freezer as it makes me eat them slower.)

Green Smoothie

A great way to start the day or top off a workout! You can vary the fruit used.

Recipe serves: 1

Ingredients:

- 1 cup pure water
- 1 banana
- 1 cup kale or spinach
- 1 cup frozen berries
- 3-4 Medjool dates
- 1 tablespoon chia seeds or ground flaxseeds
- Optional protein choices: hemp protein, 3 ounces of tofu, or vegan protein powder (watch for sugar content – choose one with few ingredients such as Orgain Simple)

Directions:

1. Blend together in a blender until smooth and enjoy!

Tofu Scramble

This is one of my favorite things to eat for breakfast, or any-time. To make it southwestern, wrap in a whole-grain tortilla and add guacamole and salsa.

Recipe serves: 4

Ingredients:

- 16-ounce block of high protein tofu, mashed
- 1 red, green, or yellow bell pepper, chopped
- 1 medium onion, diced
- 4 cloves garlic, chopped
- ½-1 cup nutritional yeast
- 2 tablespoons low-sodium tamari
- 1 teaspoon turmeric powder

Directions:

1. Sautee onion, pepper, and garlic in a little water or veg-etable broth.
2. Add the remaining ingredients and cook on low for 15 minutes to allow the flavors to soak into the tofu.
3. Serve in a tortilla or with some whole-grain bread and hash brown potatoes.

Dr. Deb's Gluten-Free Amazing Waffles

These are a crowd favorite and can be made ahead and frozen. Enjoy them the traditional way with pure maple syrup and fruit or smeared with peanut butter and banana.

Recipe serves: 12

Ingredients:

- 4 cups plant-based milk
- ¼ cup chia seeds, soaked in 2 cups water for 3 minutes
- 2 cups GF oats
- 2 cups millet flour
- 2 cups buckwheat flour
- 1 teaspoon sea salt
- 4 teaspoons non-aluminum baking powder

Directions:

1. Blend soaked chia seeds and water with the plant-based milk.
2. Add oats and baking powder and blend well.
3. Mix remaining ingredients in a large bowl.
4. Pour blended wet mixture into dry mixture and mix well.
5. Bake in waffle maker for 9 minutes (time may vary depending on waffle maker).
6. Serve immediately or cool on cooling rack and freeze in gallon freezer bags to pop in the toaster when needed.

Gaga's Granola

Most of my grandkids call me Gaga, hence the name of this recipe. This granola is great added to a smoothie bowl, topped over fresh fruit, or eaten alone as a snack.

Recipe serves: 12

Ingredients:

- 4 cups rolled oats
- 1 cup walnuts, chopped
- ½ cup raw sunflower seeds
- 1 cup raisins
- ½ cups dates, chopped
- 1 teaspoon cinnamon
- ¼ cups pure maple syrup

Directions:

1. Preheat oven to 275°.
2. Combine the oats, walnuts, and sunflower seeds and spread evenly on a baking sheet.
3. Bake for 15 minutes.
4. Stir the mixture and again spread out evenly on sheet. Bake another 15 minutes.
5. Remove from oven and place in a non-plastic bowl. Add remaining ingredients except the maple syrup and mix well.
6. Add the maple syrup and mix well.
7. Allow to cool and store in an airtight container.

Banana Peanut Butter Muffins

I modified a recipe I found and came up with this recipe which is delicious. You can make them gluten-free or not.

Recipe serves: 12

Ingredients:

- 1 ¾ cups Bob's Red Mill Gluten-free 1 to 1 Baking Flour, or whole-wheat pastry flour
- ¾ cup monk fruit or coconut sugar
- 1 Tablespoon baking powder
- ½ teaspoon salt
- 1 teaspoon cinnamon
- 1 cup mashed ripe bananas (about 2 medium)
- ½ cup plant-based milk
- ½ cup peanut or almond butter
- ½ cup cacao powder (or cocoa powder)
- 2 tablespoons pure maple syrup
- Topping: 2 Tablespoons monk fruit or coconut sugar mixed with 1 teaspoon cinnamon

Directions:

1. Preheat oven to 400° and oil muffin tins.
2. Mix dry ingredients except topping ingredients together in large bowl.
3. Mix wet ingredients in smaller bowl.
4. Add wet to dry and place in 12 muffin tins.
5. Sprinkle topping on top of each muffin.
6. Bake for 20 minutes or until toothpick inserted comes out clean.

DIPS AND SAUCES RECIPES

Better Than Pimento Cheese

Being raised in Kentucky, I can tell you I loved pimento cheese. I was so excited to find this recipe that gives that yummy pimento cheese flavor without the cholesterol and harmful fat.

Recipe serves: 4

Ingredients:

- 1.5 cups raw sunflower seeds
- 1 large red-bell pepper, chopped
- 2 cloves garlic, diced
- ½ cup sesame seeds
- Juice of 1 lemon
- 1 teaspoon tamari

Directions:

1. Sauté pepper and garlic in water or vegetable broth.
2. Place in food processor with the remaining ingredients.
3. Blend until very smooth adding water if necessary.
4. Serve with crudités and crackers, on a sandwich, or in a wrap.

Almond Herb Dip

Such a delicious dip that is always a crowd pleaser!

Recipe serves: 4

Ingredients:

- 1 cup raw almonds, soaked for 2 hours
- 1 bulb (not clove) garlic, roasted
- ¼ cup nutritional yeast
- 2 tablespoons tamari
- Juice of 1 lemon
- 1 handful fresh herbs of choice

Directions:

1. Drain and rinse almonds.
2. Blend all ingredients in a food process until smooth.
3. Serve with crudités and crackers, on a sandwich, or in a wrap.

Artichoke Pesto

Artichokes have many health benefits. I like to serve this as a dip or over pasta. Artichokes can be used in recipes to thicken and smooth, instead of oil.

Recipe serves: 4

Ingredients:

- 15-ounce can artichoke hearts in water, drained
- 4 cloves garlic, raw or roasted
- 1 bunch basil or cilantro
- ¼ cup lemon juice
- 1 cup walnuts
- Salt and pepper to taste

Directions:

1. Blend all ingredients in food processor or blender until smooth.

Enrique's Cilantro Sauce

This is such a great sauce to pour over potatoes, rice, veggies, whatever. So delicious and nutritious created by my son, Enrique.

Recipe serves: 6-8

Ingredients:

- 1 bunch cilantro
- 4 cloves garlic, raw or roasted
- 8 ounces vegan cream cheese, I prefer Violife brand
- Juice of 1 lime
- 1 serrano or jalapeño pepper, optional for those that like spice
- 2-3 ounces unsweetened plant-based milk of choice
- Salt and pepper to taste

Directions:

1. Blend all ingredients in food processor or blender until smooth.

Cashew Cheeze

This cheese can be used for homemade pizza, lasagna, or as a yummy dip for veggies.

Ingredients:

- 2 cups raw cashews, soaked for 2-4 hours
- 2 cloves raw garlic
- Juice of 1 lemon
- Handful of fresh basil, or 1 tablespoon dried basil
- Water to get to proper consistency (depends on what you are using it for)
- Salt and pepper to taste

Directions:

1. Drain cashews and add to food processor with remaining ingredients.
2. Blend and add water as needed to get a smooth consistency.

Vegan Rotel Dip

People will not be able to tell the difference in this vegan version of the crowd favorite. Serve warm at your next party and people will love it.

Ingredients:

- 8-ounce package vegan cream cheese (I prefer Violife or Miyoko brands)
- 1 can organic Rotel chilis and tomatoes
- 1 medium onion, chopped
- 3 cloves garlic, minced
- 1 box tofu crumbles (or Gardein ground, Beyond ground, etc.)
- Organic tortilla chips

Directions:

1. Spray oil a skillet and sauté tofu crumbles, onion, and garlic until browned.
2. Add with remaining ingredients in a crock pot or Instant pot on slow cook mode.
3. Heat to bubbling. Reduce heat and simmer.
4. Keep hot while serving. Serve with tortilla chips.

Wise and Otherwise Dip

I created this dip in honor of my friend, Sue Wise, after she passed away. It is also named after a great game called Wise and Otherwise, which I highly recommend. You can use this as a dip or a sauce on pasta, etc.

Recipe serves: 4

Ingredients:

- 1 small yellow or red bell pepper, coarsely chopped
- 1 bulb garlic, peeled and chopped
- 1/3 cup water
- ¼ cup lemon juice (about 1.5 lemons)
- 1 can artichoke hearts, drained
- ½ teaspoon kelp, optional
- ½ teaspoon dulse, optional
- 1 teaspoon salt
- ½ teaspoon cayenne pepper
- ¼ cup raw sesame seeds
- ½ cup raw sunflower seeds
- ½ cup raw pumpkin seeds
- Ground black pepper to taste

Directions:

1. Spray oil a skillet and sauté bell pepper and garlic until soft.
2. Add to remaining ingredients in a food process and process until smooth.
3. Chill before serving with raw veggies and crackers.

Raw Hummus

This is amazingly good in place of traditional hummus. Serve with raw veggies, crackers, or on a wrap.

Recipe serves: 4-6

Ingredients:

- 1 large zucchini
- ½ cup raw almond butter or tahini
- 2 tablespoons extra virgin olive oil
- 2 tablespoons lemon juice
- 1 large clove garlic
- Pinch of cayenne (optional)
- Sprinkle of paprika
- Salt and black pepper to taste

Directions:

1. Place all ingredients in a food processor and process until smooth.
2. Chill before serving.

Roasted Eggplant Dip

Yummy dip incorporating eggplant.

Recipe serves: 4-6

Ingredients:

- 4 long Japanese eggplant
- 1 cup almonds or cashews, soaked for several hours
- ½ cup Veganaise (or other vegan mayo)
- 2 tablespoons lemon juice
- 1 large clove garlic
- 1 tablespoon tamari
- Salt and ground black pepper to taste

Directions:

1. Roast eggplant whole in 375° oven for 20 minutes or until soft.
2. Cut and scoop out the middle and place in a food processor. Discard skins.
3. Add remaining ingredients and process until smooth.
4. May serve warm or chilled. This is great in a wrap with lettuce, tomatoes, and chopped onions.

Chickpea of the Sea Spread

Reminiscent of tuna salad but without the mercury! Remember, beans are a superfood that we should consume daily to live in peak health. They are full of protein, fiber, and nutrients. **You can substitute a package of tofu for the beans in this recipe for an eggless salad that is also delicious.** Enjoy this spread on a sandwich, wrap, or as a dip.

Recipe serves: 4

Ingredients:

- 15-ounce can of chickpeas (also known as garbanzo beans), drained
- ½ cup Veganaise or other vegan mayo
- 2 tablespoons mustard of choice
- 1 cup celery, diced
- 2 tablespoons sweet pickle relish
- ¼ cup sweet onion, diced
- 1 teaspoon garlic powder
- Salt and pepper to taste

Directions:

1. Mash chickpeas by hand or in a food processor.
2. Add remaining ingredients and mix well.

SALAD RECIPES

Thai Crunch Salad

I love Thai food! Thai restaurants are usually great options for vegans. This salad is delicious and nutritious.

Recipe serves: 6

Dressing Ingredients:

- ¼ cup smooth no-sugar peanut butter
- 2 tablespoons rice vinegar
- 2 tablespoons lime juice
- 1 tablespoon tamari
- 3 Medjool dates
- 2 cloves of raw garlic
- ½ inch piece of peeled ginger
- ¼ teaspoon crushed red pepper flakes
- 2 tablespoons fresh cilantro

Salad Ingredients:

- 4 cups finely chopped cabbage
- 1 cup shredded carrots
- 1 red bell pepper, thinly sliced
- 1 small English cucumber, chopped
- 2 medium scallions, chopped

Directions:

1. Blend dressing in blender until smooth.
2. Combine salad ingredients in a large bowl.
3. Add dressing and mix well.
4. May top with raw sesame seeds.

Spinach Strawberry Salad

This recipe is always a crowd pleaser. Full of phytonutrients, it contains some of the healthiest produce on the planet.

Recipe serves: 6

Dressing Ingredients:

- ½ mashed avocado or ¼ cup extra virgin olive oil
- 1/3 cup date sugar or monk fruit sweetener
- ¼ cup apple cider vinegar
- 1 clove raw garlic
- Salt and pepper to taste

Salad Ingredients:

- 6 cups torn spinach or mixed greens
- 2.5 cups sliced strawberries
- ½ cup walnuts, chopped
- 1 cup Violife shredded mozzarella cheese, or another vegan mozzarella, optional

Directions:

1. Blend dressing together.
2. Add to salad and mix well right before serving.

Quinoa Market Salad

Combining the protein and nutrition of the ancient grain of quinoa with some good veggies is satisfying and healthy.

Recipe serves: 6

Ingredients:

- 2 cups quinoa, cooked according to directions
- 4 cups raw vegetables of choice
- Fresh herbs of choice
- ¼ cup hemp hearts
- Juice of 1 lemon or lime, or 2 tablespoons apple cider vinegar
- 2 cloves raw or roasted garlic, minced, or 1 teaspoon garlic powder
- Salt and pepper to taste

Directions:

1. Cook quinoa according to directions and allow to cool.
2. Mix in a large bowl with the other ingredients.
3. Chill before serving.

Kale Avocado Salad

This salad is a yummy way to get the abundant nutrients of kale into your diet.

Recipe serves: 6

Ingredients:

- 1 bunch kale, chopped
- ½ cup fruit juice-sweetened dried cranberries
- 2 scallions including the green part, chopped
- ¼ cup hemp hearts
- 4 pieces hearts of palm, chopped
- Bragg's Braggberry dressing
- Salt and pepper to taste

Directions:

1. Put chopped kale in large bowl and sprinkle a bit of salt on top.
2. Add the dressing.
3. Massage the kale with your hands to make kale more tender.
4. Add the remaining ingredients and mix well.

Beet Carrot Slaw

This is a colorful slaw full of nutrient-dense produce.

Recipe serves: 4

Ingredients:

- 2 medium beets, shredded
- 1 large carrot, shredded
- 1 medium apple, shredded
- ¼ cup raisins
- ¼ cup walnut pieces
- ½ cup Veganaise (or another vegan mayo)
- 2 tablespoons apple cider vinegar
- 2 tablespoons maple syrup or honey
- Salt and pepper to taste

Directions:

1. Place beets, carrot, apple, raisins, and walnuts in a bowl. Mix well.
2. Combine remaining ingredients and add to bowl.
3. Mix well and serve alone or on top of mixed greens.

Quinoa Tabouli

My gluten-free version of the traditional Mediterranean salad. Very satisfying and healthy!

Recipe serves: 4

Dressing Ingredients:

- 1 cup quinoa, cooked according to directions, and cooled
- 1 large clove garlic, minced
- 1-2 cups tomatoes, chopped
- 1 bunch parsley, chopped finely
- 2 tablespoons extra-virgin olive oil
- Juice from ½ large lemon
- 1 teaspoon sea salt

Directions:

1. Add all ingredients in a large bowl and mix well.
2. Allow to chill for one hour.
3. Serve over a bed of shredded lettuce or alone.

APPETIZERS AND SIDE DISH RECIPES

Southwestern Pinwheels

This is a delicious recipe and a great thing to take to potlucks or parties. Always a crowd pleaser!

Recipe serves: 20

Ingredients:

- 8-ounces vegan cream cheese, softened (I prefer Violife or Miyoko's)
- ½ cup shredded vegan cheddar-style cheese (I prefer Violife)
- 2 green onions including the green part, thinly sliced
- 1 tablespoon canned chipotle chilies in adobe sauce, chopped (use this only if you like spicy)
- 4 tablespoon chunky salsa
- 4 tablespoons cilantro, chopped
- 1 teaspoon cumin
- Spinach
- 10-inch whole-grain or GF tortillas
- Cilantro strips for garnish

Directions:

1. Mix all ingredients except spinach, tortillas, and cilantro strips in a bowl. Mix well.
2. Spread over tortillas and add a cilantro strip.
3. Roll and cut in 1-inch pieces. Line on a plate with a bowl of extra salsa.

Garlic Mashed Sweet Potatoes

Very yummy and great for the holidays!

Recipe serves: 4

Ingredients:

- 2 large sweet potatoes, peeled and cut in thick slices
- 1 bulb (not clove) garlic, roasted
- ½ lemon, juiced
- Salt and pepper to taste

Directions:

1. Place the sweet potatoes in a pan and cover with water. Cook until tender.
2. Cut off the bottom of the bulb of garlic. Place in aluminum foil and roast in a 400° oven for 30-40 minutes until soft. Cool and squeeze the garlic out.
3. Mash sweet potatoes with the remaining ingredients including a bit of cooking water reserved from the potatoes.

Spicy Peanut Butter Tofu with Sriracha

This is one of my favorites!

Recipe serves: 4

Ingredients:

- 16-ounce block of firm or extra firm tofu (usually labeled high protein)
- 1 tablespoon coconut oil

Sauce Ingredients:

- 3 tablespoons tamari
- 3 tablespoons apple cider or rice vinegar
- 2 tablespoons smooth peanut butter
- 1 tablespoon pure maple syrup
- 2 tablespoons vegetable broth or water
- 1 tablespoon sriracha (for those who like heat)

Directions:

1. Drain and cube tofu. Press in paper towels to remove any water.
2. Heat oil in skillet and fry the tofu until crispy and golden. For an oil-free version, cook on 300° in an air fryer until crispy (about 10-20 minutes).
3. Meanwhile place all sauce ingredients in a jar and shake well to combine.
4. Pour sauce over tofu and serve. Can be served over a bed of rice or as an appetizer.

SOUP RECIPES

West African Vegan Winter Soup

I was inspired to create this after tasting something similar in a café here in town. My husband and I both love this soup!

Recipe serves: 6

Ingredients:

- 1 medium onion, diced
- 1 medium carrot, chopped
- 3 stalks celery, diced
- 2 large sweet potatoes, peeled and chopped
- 1 medium yellow pepper, diced
- 2 garlic cloves, minced
- ½ cup white wine, or water
- 20 ounces crushed tomatoes
- 2 cups vegetable broth
- 24 ounces water
- 3 cups chopped kale
- ½ cup chopped cilantro
- 1 tablespoon turmeric powder
- 1 tablespoon diced fresh ginger, or 1 teaspoon powdered ginger
- 1 cup peanut butter (or almond butter)
- Salt and pepper to taste
- Chopped cilantro for garnish

Directions:

1. Place all vegetables in white wine or water and sauté for 10 minutes.
2. Add tomatoes, vegetable broth, and water and simmer for 20 minutes.

3. Once vegetables are soft, remove 2 cups and blend with peanut butter.
4. Return to soup and mix well. Serve with chopped cilantro.

Simple Butternut Squash Soup

This was shared with me from my sweet Cuban friend, Isabel. It is super easy, delicious, and nutritious!

Recipe serves: 4

Ingredients:

- 1 medium butternut squash, peeled and cubed
- 1 large onion, chopped
- 1 bulb garlic, roasted
- 1 cup cashews, raw or roasted
- 2 tablespoons Tamari
- Garlic powder
- Chili powder
- 1 32-ounce container organic low-sodium vege-table broth
- Chopped cilantro for garnish

Directions:

1. Spray baking sheet with oil and add butternut squash in a single layer.
2. Bake in 350° oven or air fryer until soft.
3. Coat the cashews with tamari. Sprinkle with garlic powder and chili powder. Bake in 250° oven for 20 minutes.
4. Add all ingredients to blender and blend until smooth. Add more water if needed.
5. Serve with chopped cilantro or other herb of choice.

August Summer Soup

I created this on 8/1/07 from things I had in the house. One of the best soups ever in my opinion. Soup and salad are such a great meal anytime! It's a great idea to make a big batch of soup on the weekend to enjoy during the week when you don't have a lot of time to cook.

Recipe serves: 4

Ingredients:

- 1 large onion, diced
- 1 jalapeño, halved with seeds removed (optional for those who like a little heat)
- 1 large yellow squash, diced
- 1 medium ripe tomato, diced
- 2 cloves garlic, minced
- 1 stalk broccoli, chopped
- 15-ounce can pinto beans
- ¾ cup refried beans
- ½ teaspoon cumin
- 1 teaspoon chili powder
- 1 cup cooked quinoa
- Several cups water or vegetable broth
- Salt and pepper to taste

Directions:

1. Sauté garlic and onion in a little water or vegetable broth until onions are translucent.
2. Add remaining ingredients and bring to a boil. Lower heat and simmer for 15-30 minutes or until veggies are tender.

Creamy Broccoli Soup

This is so delicious and nutritious. Remember broccoli is the number one food to fight cancer.

Recipe serves: 6

Ingredients:

- 1 cup onion, diced
- 1 tablespoon oil
- 2 pounds fresh or frozen broccoli
- ¾ cup celery, chopped
- 3 cloves garlic, minced
- 1 teaspoon dried thyme
- 1.5 tablespoons fresh ginger, minced (or 1 teaspoon dried ginger)
- 3.5 cups plain plant-based milk, or water
- 4 cups water
- 3 teaspoons arrowroot powder dissolved in 3 tablespoons of water
- 1 tablespoon fresh lemon or lime juice
- Salt and pepper to taste

Directions:

1. Separate broccoli into stems and florets.
2. Peel and slice stems into small thin pieces.
3. Chop florets.
4. Add 3.5 cups plant-based milk or water to pan. Add ½ broccoli stems and a pinch of salt. Bring to a simmer over medium heat. Reduce heat to low and cook for 5 minutes.
5. Meanwhile, in a large pot, heat oil over medium heat. Add remaining broccoli stems, onion, celery, ginger, garlic, and thyme. Cook over medium heat for 10 minutes, stirring.

6. Add florets and 4 cups water and stir well. Bring to simmer over medium heat.
7. Reduce to low and cook for 10 minutes.
8. Stir in arrowroot mixture and cook for 8 minutes, stirring occasionally.
9. Blend the broccoli liquid mixture from step 4 and add to pot. Add salt and pepper to taste and stir well. Serve with lemon or lime juice.

Creamy Tomato Veggie Soup

I created this recipe for a business potluck I hosted. It was a big hit!

Recipe serves: 8

Ingredients:

- 1 large onion, diced
- ½ head cauliflower, chopped
- 2 large carrots, sliced
- ½ head cabbage, chopped
- 1 large zucchini, sliced
- 3 cloves garlic, minced, or 1 tablespoon dried garlic powder
- 45 ounces pureed jarred tomatoes
- 5 cups water
- 1 teaspoon dried basil
- 1 tablespoon no-salt herb mix
- 1 bay leaf
- 15-ounce can coconut milk
- Salt and pepper to taste

Directions:

1. Spray large soup pan with oil. Start adding vegetables one by one and sauté.
2. Add remaining ingredients except coconut milk and bring to a simmer over medium heat.
3. Simmer on medium-low for 30 minutes or until veggies are tender.
4. Scoop out several cups of vegetables and add to blender with the coconut milk. Blend until smooth.
5. Add blended mixture back to soup and mix well.

Creamy Quinoato Soup

My hubby named this soup, and it is delicious. Full of great quality plant protein and phytonutrients.

Recipe serves: 4

Ingredients:

- 1 tablespoon extra-virgin olive oil
- 1 large onion, diced
- 2 medium carrots, sliced
- 1 bay leaf
- 5 Roma tomatoes, halved
- 2 cups jarred diced tomatoes
- 3 cups water
- 1 teaspoon dried basil
- ½ cup vegan sour cream (my favorite is Forager)
- ¾ cup uncooked quinoa
- Salt and pepper to taste

Directions:

1. Sauté onion and tomatoes in oil or water.
2. Add remaining ingredients except sour cream and bring to a simmer over a medium heat.
3. Cook for an hour, stirring occasionally.
4. Remove the Roma tomatoes and blend with the sour cream. Add back and stir well.

Fantastic Fall Bisque

A wonderful soup to warm the bones on a chilly night.

Recipe serves: 4

Ingredients:

- 1 medium butternut squash, peeled and cubed
- 12 ounces fingerling potatoes
- 2 large stalks celery, diced
- 1 large onion, diced
- ½ bunch kale, chopped
- 1 cup fresh dill, parsley, and cilantro (or other herbs of choice)
- 1 clove garlic, minced
- 1 can coconut milk
- Salt and pepper to taste

Directions:

1. Add all ingredients except coconut milk to soup pot.
2. Cover with water and bring to a simmer over medium heat.
3. Lower heat and cook until tender (about 30 minutes).
4. Add coconut milk and blend the soup with an immersion blender or add to a blender with the coconut milk and blend until smooth.

Fall Mushroom Bisque

If you like mushrooms, you will enjoy this yummy soup. Mushrooms are great for your health.

Recipe serves: 4

Ingredients:

- 1 large pack baby portabella mushrooms (2 pints)
- 1 large sweet onion, diced
- 2 tablespoons coconut oil
- 2 cloves garlic, minced
- 1 teaspoon dried thyme
- ¼ cup brandy, or cooking wine
- 3.5 cups low-sodium vegetable broth, or water
- 1 cup plain plant-based milk
- Salt and pepper to taste

Directions:

1. Chop onions and mushrooms very finely in food processor.
2. Sauté onions, garlic, and thyme in oil (or water for oil-free cooking) in soup pan.
3. Add brandy and mushrooms and sauté for 10 minutes.
4. Add broth or water and cook for 10 minutes.
5. Blend ¾ cup soup with milk in blender and add back to soup. Mix well.

Summer Gazpacho

This is so refreshing in the summertime when fresh produce is so readily available.

Recipe serves: 4

Ingredients:

- 1 large cucumber
- 1 large stalk celery
- 8 ounces fresh tomatoes
- 1 clove garlic
- 1 tablespoon lemon or lime juice
- ½ teaspoon dried cumin
- Salt and pepper to taste

Directions:

1. Add all ingredients to blender and blend until smooth.
2. May serve with a sprinkle of cayenne if you like spicy foods. Also, may top with raw or roasted pumpkin seeds.

In a Pinch Soup

This is super easy for a quick meal. It is great pared with a nice salad.

Recipe serves: 4

Ingredients:

- 24-ounce jar pureed tomatoes (I like Bionaturae brand)
- 2 cups chopped cauliflower
- 1 stalk celery, chopped
- 4 medium potatoes, peeled and chopped
- 1 clove garlic, minced
- 1 can pinto beans
- 1 tablespoon chili powder
- 1 can coconut milk
- Salt and pepper to taste

Directions:

1. Sauté cauliflower, celery, garlic, and potatoes in vegetable broth or water for 10 minutes.
2. Add remaining ingredients except coconut milk and bring to a simmer over medium heat.
3. Reduce heat and simmer for 30 minutes until veggies are tender.
4. Add coconut milk 5 minutes prior to serving. Mix well.

ENTRÉE RECIPES

Lentil Shepherd's Pie

This recipe is contributed by Carol Watson, ND, and is so delicious and satisfying! Check out her info at www.TcDrCarol.com.

Recipe serves: 6

Ingredients:

- 1 cup onion, diced
- 1 cup carrot, diced
- ½ cup celery, diced
- ½ cup green beans, roughly chopped
- 1 cup diced parsnip, or potato
- 2 large cloves garlic, minced
- 4 cups vegetable broth
- ½ cup organic red wine, optional
- 1 cup uncooked green lentils, rinsed and drained
- 1 teaspoon dried sage
- 2 teaspoons dried thyme
- 2 tablespoons non-GMO arrowroot or flour to thicken
- Salt and pepper to taste

Topping Ingredients:

- 1 head cauliflower
- 2 medium sweet potatoes
- 1/3 cup plain plant-based milk
- 3-4 tablespoons Earth Balance (or any plant-based butter substitute)

Directions:

1. In a large pot over medium heat, sauté all veggies and garlic for about 7 minutes, or until onions are translucent and veggies are slightly tender.
2. Add salt and pepper to taste.
3. Add vegetable broth, wine, lentils, thyme and sage. Bring to a boil, reduce heat, and let simmer for 35- 40 minutes, or until lentils are tender.
4. Gradually stir arrowroot powder or flour into mixture and keep gently stirring until thickened.
5. Preheat oven to 425°.
6. Meanwhile, steam cauliflower and sweet potatoes until fork tender. Drain water. Add plant-based milk and buttery spread and mash with a fork. Add salt and pepper to taste.
7. Transfer lentil mixture to a 9x13 baking dish. Carefully spread mashed cauliflower evenly over top. Bake at 425° for 10 minutes and then transfer to under the broiler for 5 minutes, or until a nice lightly browned/ golden color. Remove from oven and let cool briefly before serving.

Easy Pad Thai

This is an easy and delicious version of Pad Thai minus the egg.

Recipe serves: 4

Ingredients:

- 1 package pad Thai noodles
- 3 tablespoons tamari
- 3 tablespoons apple cider or rice vinegar
- 2 tablespoons smooth peanut butter
- 1 tablespoon maple syrup
- 2 tablespoons vegetable broth or water
- 1 tablespoon sriracha (for those who like heat)

Directions:

1. Cook noodles according to package directions.
2. Combine the remaining ingredients in a jar and shake well. Pour over noodles.
3. You may top Pad Thai with chopped peanuts, chopped cilantro, and chopped green onions for an authentic Thai experience.

Lentil Loaf

This recipe is contributed by Carol Watson, ND, and is great at holidays or anytime you want some comfort food! Check out her info at www.TcDrCarol.com.

Recipe serves: 6

Ingredients:

- 2 cups cooked green lentils
- 1 cup shredded medium potato (may substitute sweet potato)
- 1 cup celery, diced
- 1 clove garlic, minced
- 1 tablespoon olive oil, or vegetable broth
- 1 cup gluten-free oats
- ½ cup fresh parsley, chopped
- 1 cup tomato puree
- 1 tablespoon ground flaxseeds
- 2 tablespoons warm water
- 1 tablespoon fresh thyme, chopped, or 1 teaspoon dried
- 1 tablespoon fresh rosemary, chopped, or 1 teaspoon dried
- Salt and pepper to taste

Glaze Ingredients:

- ¼ cup organic ketchup
- ¼ teaspoon smoked paprika
- 2 tablespoons balsamic vinegar
- 1 tablespoon pure maple syrup

Directions:

1. Preheat oven to 350°.
2. Mix the ground flaxseeds and warm water and set aside.
3. Sauté the onion and celery in the oil or vegetable broth until onion is translucent.
4. Add the garlic and sauté another few minutes. Remove from heat.
5. Combine all the loaf ingredients, including the flax-seed and water mixture, in a large bowl. Add salt and pepper to taste.
6. Turn the loaf mixture into a lightly greased loaf pan.
7. In a small bowl mix the glaze ingredients and brush on the top of the loaf.
8. Bake for 50 minutes. Allow to cool for 10 minutes before serving.

Tempeh Sloppy Joes

This recipe is contributed by Carol Watson, ND, and is great served on whole-grain buns or bread. Check out her info at www.TcDrCarol.com.

Recipe serves: 6

Ingredients:

- 8-oz package of tempeh, crumbled
- 1 large onion, diced
- 1 red pepper, diced
- 2 cloves garlic, minced
- 15-oz jar organic tomatoes
- 1 tablespoon extra-virgin olive oil
- 1 teaspoon chili powder, or more to taste
- 1 teaspoon ground cumin
- 1 teaspoon dried mustard powder
- 2 tablespoons sweetener of choice – coconut sugar, pure maple syrup, etc.
- 1/8 teaspoon dried celery seed
- 1 tablespoon ACV (apple cider vinegar)
- Salt and pepper to taste

Directions:

1. Heat oil in a heavy-duty sauté pan on medium-high. Add tempeh.
2. Add onions when tempeh is a golden color.
3. When onions become translucent, add the remaining ingredients.
4. After 2 minutes, reduce heat to medium and cook, stirring occasionally, for 10 minutes.

Sloppy Janes

Another version of a sloppy Joe that I like using tofu instead of tempeh.

Recipe serves: 6

Ingredients:

- 16-oz package high-protein tofu, crumbled
- 28-ounce jar of tomatoes
- 2 cloves garlic, minced
- 2-4 tablespoons chili powder
- 1 medium onion, diced
- 1 medium green pepper, diced
- ¼ cup ketchup
- ¼ cup mustard of choice
- 2 tablespoons tamari
- Salt and pepper to taste

Directions:

1. Sauté onion and pepper in a small amount of vegetable broth.
2. Add tofu to the vegetables.
3. Add remaining ingredients and simmer for 30 minutes.
4. Enjoy on a toasted bun or in a whole-grain tortilla.

Deb's Famous Pizza

Everyone that tastes this pizza loves it, even meat and cheese lovers. My grandkids say it is their favorite pizza, which is saying a lot! The dough recipe is from the back of the Jovial all-purpose flour bag.

Recipe serves: 8

Crust Ingredients:

- 1 ¼ cups water
- 3 tablespoons extra virgin olive oil
- 2 teaspoons salt
- 1 teaspoon sugar
- 1 teaspoon active dry yeast
- 5 cups all-purpose Einkorn flour

Pizza Ingredients:

- Chopped veggies of choice: onion, pepper, mushrooms, zucchini, olives, etc.
- 1 jar marinara sauce
- 1 batch cashew cheeze (recipe in Dips and Sauces section)

Directions:

1. Put all crust ingredients in a bread maker and use the dough mode. Once dough is ready, remove from bread maker and flatten on an oiled cookie sheet or pizza stone (if using pizza stone, heat ahead of time.) **If you don't have a bread maker, simply follow the directions on the back of the bag of flour.** Cover and allow to sit for 30 minutes. It should rise a bit. If you are in a hurry, you can skip this step. It will still rise in the oven. This recipe can be used as a thicker crust using one

cookie sheet, or you can make it thinner using two cookie sheets.

2. Preheat oven to 425°. Bake dough for 10 minutes. Remove from oven.
3. Spread cashew cheeze over entire dough using a spatula.
4. Spread marinara sauce over the cheeze. Add generous toppings of choice.
5. Bake for 15-20 minutes until crust is a perfect crispiness. Remove from oven, slice, and enjoy.

Healthy Vegan Mac-n-Cheeze

Mac-n-cheese is always a hit, especially with kids. This is a healthy version full of phytonutrients, yet it still satisfies the palette!

Recipe serves: 6

Ingredients:

- 1 medium butternut squash, peeled and cut in 2-inch cubes
- ¼ cup miso
- ¼ cup hot water
- ¼ cup nutritional yeast flakes
- 3 tablespoons Dijon mustard
- 2 tablespoons raw tahini
- 3 tablespoons tamari
- 1-pound eggless elbow macaroni
- ½ cup breadcrumbs (optional)
- Salt and pepper to taste

Directions:

1. Preheat oven to 350°.
2. Spray oil a 1.5-quart baking dish.
3. Cook pasta according to directions. Drain.
4. Steam butternut squash until tender, approximately 15-20 minutes.
5. Put ½ the butternut squash in a blender with the miso, hot water, nutritional yeast, mustard, tahini, and tamari. Blend until smooth.
6. Add remaining ½ of butternut squash, blended mixture, pasta, salt and pepper in the baking dish. Mix well.
7. Top with breadcrumbs and bake for 20 minutes.

Tofu Pot Pie

This is one of my favorite recipes and is always a crowd pleaser, even amongst meat eaters. It's a bit labor intensive but so worth the effort. I don't typically cook with much oil but with this recipe, I splurge and use the oil. If you are reversing heart disease, avoid the oil and use vegetable broth or water instead.

Recipe serves: 4-6

Ingredients:

- ¼ cup whole-wheat pastry flour, or flour of choice
- 1 tablespoon nutritional yeast flakes
- 1 teaspoon sea salt
- ½ teaspoon garlic powder
- 16-ounce package of high-protein tofu, cut in cubes
- 2 tablespoons coconut oil, or oil of choice
- 1 cup onions, chopped
- ½ cup celery, diced
- 2 cups frozen mixed vegetables

Gravy Ingredients:

- 1/3 cup whole-wheat pastry flour, or other flour
- 1/3 cup nutritional yeast flakes
- ¼ cup coconut oil
- 2 cups water
- 1 tablespoon tamari

Gravy Directions:

1. Toast the flour in a skillet until fragrant.
2. Add the nutritional yeast and oil and stir well.
3. Slowly add the water stirring constantly.
4. Add the tamari and mix well. Set aside.

Directions:

1. Preheat oven to 375°.
2. Combine the flour, nutritional yeast flakes, salt, and garlic powder in a bowl.
3. Add the tofu cubes and stir to coat.
4. Heat a skillet and sauté tofu in the coconut oil until lightly browned.
5. Add the onions and celery to the pan and sauté until they are soft.
6. Add the frozen vegetables and mix well. Remove from heat.
7. Add the gravy to the mixture.
8. Place in a baking dish. Top with mashed potatoes or pie crust (see recipe in Pecan Pie recipe).
9. Bake for 30-40 minutes until bubbly.

Mexican Lasagna

A Mexican twist on an Italian favorite! Eat with guacamole, chips and salsa to make it a full Mexican meal.

Recipe serves: 6

Ingredients:

- 1 package lasagna noodles (I like Jovial brown rice lasagna)
- 2 15-ounce cans of vegan refried beans
- 1 large container salsa of choice
- 1 batch of cashew cheeze (recipe in Dips and Sauces), or Violife cheddar shreds
- Vegetables of choice (as many as you want) – I use frozen corn, mushrooms, sauteed bell peppers, and sliced carrots

Directions:

1. Place plenty of salsa on the bottom of a lasagna pan to cover it.
2. Layer noodles (not necessary to pre-cook), refried beans, cheese, veggies and salsa.
3. Finish with a good layer of salsa so noodles will cook.
4. Cover & bake on 350° for 45 minutes.

DESSERT RECIPES

Grain-Free Peanut Butter Cookies

These cookies are surprisingly good and include the benefit of legumes. They are very moist!

Recipe serves: 12

Ingredients:

- ½ cup plus 2 tablespoons peanut butter
- ½ cup pure maple syrup
- 15-ounce can cannellini beans, drained
- 1 teaspoon non-aluminum baking powder
- ½ cup vegan chocolate chips

Directions:

1. Preheat oven to 350°.
2. Line a cookie sheet with parchment paper.
3. Place beans in a bowl and mash with a fork.
4. Add remaining ingredients and stir.
5. Drop by heaping teaspoon onto cookie sheet.
6. Bake for 30 minutes until slightly brown.
7. Turn cookies over and bake another 10 minutes.
8. Cool and enjoy!

Caramel Apple Crunch

A delicious and nutritious dessert!

Recipe serves: 4-6

Ingredients:

- 1 cup rolled oats
- ½ cup coconut sugar or monk fruit sweetener
- ½ cup flour of choice
- 1 teaspoon cinnamon
- ¼ teaspoon salt
- 3 medium apples, cored and chopped in pieces
- ½ cup applesauce
- 1/3 cup raisins or dried mulberries

Directions:

1. Preheat oven to 350°.
2. In a medium bowl combine the oats, sweetener, flour, cinnamon, and salt.
3. Stir in the applesauce and mix until mixture is moist.
4. Place the apples and raisins in a 9-inch square baking dish.
5. Sprinkle with the oat mixture.
6. Bake for 35 minutes until the apples are tender. Serve warm with some optional plant-based ice cream. So yummy!

Almond Joy Drops

A great alternative to the candy that bears a similar name.

Recipe serves: 30

Ingredients:

- 1 cup almonds, roughly chopped
- 1 bag vegan chocolate chips (I prefer Lily's stevia sweetened or Enjoy Life)
- ¼ cup maple syrup
- 1 tablespoon vanilla
- ½ cup plant-based milk
- 1 ½ cup unsweetened coconut

Directions:

1. Melt chocolate chips over low heat on stove.
2. Add remaining ingredients and mix well.
3. Remove from heat and drop teaspoonfuls onto wax paper.
4. Refrigerate. Store in airtight container in the refrigerator.

Best-Ever Pecan Pie

This pie is one of the best holiday recipes ever. I won the recipe contest at a vegan potluck I attended a few years ago with this pie. You can use walnuts instead of pecans if you'd like. Either works well!

Recipe serves: 8

Ingredients:

- 3/4 cup pure maple syrup
- 1/2 teaspoon ground cinnamon
- 1 tablespoon arrowroot powder
- 2 tablespoons raw tahini
- 2 ½ cups pecan or walnut halves

Crust Ingredients:

- 1.5 cups gluten-free flour blend or whole wheat pastry flour
- 1/2 tsp salt
- 1/4–1/2 cup plant-based milk

Crust Directions:

1. Preheat oven to 350°.
2. Spray pie pan with oil.
3. Combine all ingredients into bowl.
4. Press into pie pan.
5. Poke with a fork several times on bottom and sides of crust.
6. Bake in oven for 15 minutes before filling.

Pie Directions:

1. Put the maple syrup, cinnamon, arrowroot, and tahini in a food processor and process until smooth. Add the pecans and pulse several times to coarsely chop the nuts.
2. Pour the filling into the baked pie shell.
3. Bake about 25 to 30 minutes until the filling is bubbly, and the top is evenly browned. It will still seem a bit wet but will firm up when cooled.
4. Cool completely before serving.

Perfect Pumpkin Muffins

If you are like me and love everything pumpkin, you will love these muffins.

Recipe serves: 12

Ingredients:

- 15-ounce can of organic pumpkin puree
- 1 cup plant-based milk of choice
- 2/3 cup organic applesauce
- 4 teaspoons aluminum-free baking powder
- 1 teaspoon baking soda
- 3 cups organic millet flour, or whole-wheat pastry flour for a non-GF version
- 1.5 cups monk fruit sweetener
- ½ teaspoon allspice
- ½ teaspoon ground ginger
- 2 tablespoons cinnamon
- 1/2 cup vegan chocolate chips (optional)
- 1 cup chopped walnuts, optional

Directions:

1. Preheat oven to 375°.
2. Oil and flour muffin tins.
3. Place pumpkin, milk, applesauce, spices, baking powder, and baking soda in a blender and blend until smooth. Add the mixture to a bowl and mix in the flour.
4. Stir in chocolate chips and walnuts.
5. Fill muffin tins to 2/3 full.
6. Bake until a fork inserted comes out clean. It will take about 30 minutes or more, depending on your oven.

EPILOGUE

"I always get to where I'm going by
walking away from where I've been."

Winnie the Pooh

DR. CAROL WATSON returned from a conference in
April of 2014 in a body she loathed. She looked at pictures
of herself from that conference and said, "Enough!" She was
a size twenty-six and weighed 315 pounds. She has struggled with food addiction most of her life. Addiction is addiction, but one thing we all need to realize is that overcoming
a food addiction is more challenging than most addictions,
simply because you cannot abstain from the substance you are
addicted to, as people can with alcohol, drugs, etc. One must
eat in order to survive. Another thing I might note is that Carol
eats healthy. Even at that time, she was ninety-percent plant-
based, ate organic, non-GMO, etc. However, it doesn't matter
that you eat healthy if you eat way too much food. You will
still be overweight as Carol experienced. Remember, being
overweight is a health issue, not a cosmetic one.

Carol began her personal transformation in April of 2014 by
making that one decision that enough was enough. She got
to where she was going by first walking away from where she
had been. She accredits her weight loss journey to loving herself into the body she wanted. She now walks five miles a day,

and for the first time in her life, she is playing a sport—pickleball (which she loves, by the way)! She is full of energy and vitality and body confidence. She now helps other women who struggle with food addiction and body confidence.

Can you imagine how daunting the task of losing more than one-hundred pounds must feel? Carol is a fellow Naturopathic Doctor and my precious friend. We have talked every Monday morning for years. We often discussed her challenges with food addiction, and I got to witness the transformation in her. Her success is partly a result of focusing on just one day at a time, one step at a time. Carol kept her goal in mind, but instead of focusing on the one hundred thirty-pound mountain in front of her, she simply climbed one simple step at a time.

Carol's "loving herself into the body she wanted" step-by-step approach helped her lose seventy-five pounds in the first year, and one hundred thirty pounds to date. She went from a size twenty-six to a fourteen, she has more energy, improved stamina, glowing skin, and most importantly, gratitude! I am so proud of her determination to love herself into a healthier body, inch by inch, step by step![130] If she can do it, I believe anyone can if they first walk away from where they've been and follow the "inch-by-inch" philosophy I talk about here.

"Nothing is impossible, the word itself says, 'I'm possible'!"

Audrey Hepburn

---

[130] https://tcdrcarol.com/about Transformational Coaching With Dr. Carol

INCH-BY-INCH

I've introduced you to a lot of ideas that perhaps challenged your paradigms about health and vitality. You might have never heard the message that food is your best medicine, and the best foods for medicine come from the plant kingdom. Perhaps you've never heard the concept that animal products are not ideal fuel for the human body. Maybe you haven't considered that the thoughts you think and the words you speak have enormous impact on the health of your body. You may have believed that macronutrients (protein, carbohydrates, and fat) were the most important things to focus on for health, versus micronutrients.

In other words, maybe I've challenged you to think in new ways. I've covered a lot of topics in this book, and you may feel overwhelmed by the enormity of the changes in front of you. I want you to realize that it doesn't have to feel overwhelming. You can approach the process by simply starting with one change, and then moving to another once you've mastered the first thing.

However, the very first thing to realize, like Winnie the Pooh says, is that you get to where you're going by walking away from where you've been.[131] Think about the wisdom in that one statement (I love the wisdom of Pooh!). Where you are right now is the result of your daily habits to date. Getting to where you want to go (vitality, health, and longevity) requires you to walk away from the habits that have gotten you to your current state.

As the famous late personal-growth guru Jim Rohn said, "Success is nothing more than a few simple disciplines, practiced every day; while failure is simply a few errors in

---

[131]   *Christopher Robin* movie, Disney Entertainment, 2018

judgement, repeated every day."[132] Once you've made the decision to walk away from where you've been, you then start the process of habitually practicing simple disciplines that will lead to your health success.

Take a minute right now and ask yourself, "What is the mountain before *me*?"

I cannot give you the motivation to make the changes I recommend that will equip you to summit the mountain in front of you. That must come from you. Hopefully, I have nudged you just enough that the motivation is welling up within you. Hopefully you've begun to develop a vision of a healthier, more energetic tomorrow. Your future health starts right now. How you will feel five or ten years down the road begins with your next meal. You may think that it's too late to recover your health, but my belief is that if there is breath in the body, it's not too late.

YOU DO THE NATURAL; GOD ADDS THE SUPER

In the summer of 2005, my husband and I went to a personal growth camp in the mountains of British Columbia, Canada, titled Enlightened Warrior Bootcamp. It was put on by Peak Potentials and promised to be a life-altering experience. We invested $3,500 for those five days, plus airfare from Florida. We gave the experience to each other for our anniversary that year, and it was the best gift we've given each other in our thirty-one years of marriage. By far! The experience was truly supernatural.

We did the natural part: investing the money, making a commitment to finish the bootcamp no matter what (and trust me, it was far from easy), facing each day as it came, stepping out

---

[132] https://www.success.
com/15-of-jim-rohns-most-motivational-quotes/

of our comfort zones almost hourly, pushing our bodies beyond where we thought they could go, and trusting the leaders even though what they asked seemed crazy and impossible. We left with sore muscles, scratches, bruises, spider bites, and exhaustion. But we left transformed in ways beyond our wildest imaginations. That bootcamp was a kairos moment for both of us, and we have never been the same. We grew by leaps and bounds personally and spiritually that week. Outside of salvation, nothing has helped us grow more than Enlightened Warrior. They described an enlightened warrior as "one who overcomes oneself in order to better serve." I love that! I'm confident our world would be a better place if we all made that our goal. However, every single ounce of that five-day experience was hard, really hard. There were people who quit because it was so challenging. We succeeded because we were willing to do the hard natural part, and trust God to add the super. It's that divine-human partnership I mentioned earlier.

I see people who are sick with X, Y, or Z disease, and they are sitting there waiting for God to heal them. Meanwhile they continue their bad eating and lifestyle habits, not realizing that God wants them to be good stewards of their body. I'm not saying God doesn't supernaturally heal people, but for whatever reason, I just haven't seen that often. I think about the African proverb that says, "When you pray, move your feet." God wants us to do what we can to participate in our lives.

I believe that as you do the natural and begin changing your habits from destructive to healthy, God will add the super and you will experience healing and restoration—body, soul, and spirit. However, it may take time. You did not get to where you are today overnight. As I quoted earlier, it's those errors in judgement practiced daily for years that got you here. Now you begin practicing those simple disciplines today, and you practice them day in and day out, and eventually you will experience health, vitality, and happiness like never before. Trust the process. Natural healing takes time.

As a recap, here are the components of health on your HEAL compass that will lead you to longevity, health, and vitality:

- Confront the enemies of your health: you, the flock mentality, confusion (we cleared that up), the medical profession, and your priorities. Be willing to invest in your wellness now, as opposed to subsidizing your future illness.

- Live by the principle of nutrients in and toxins out. Ask, "Will this bring nutrients in and keep or get toxins out?" As Hippocrates has been credited as saying, "Let your food be your medicine and your medicine be your food."[133]

- Eat real whole plant foods full of color, enzymes, nutrients, and energy as if your life depends on it, because it does! Plant foods are the best medicine for your body, with zero side effects!

- Incorporate fasting in your life such as consuming only freshly squeezed juices, raw foods, or whole foods. Consider juicing on a regular basis. The goal of juicing and fasting is to get the nutrients in and the toxins out.

- Make more compassionate and sustainable choices and minimize or eliminate the toxins that can harm your health—such as dairy products, animal protein, sugar, and alcohol. Your body will thank you!

- Take breaks from things that can be toxic, such as junk food, television, social media, or the news.

- Win the inner game by beginning with the end in mind, reprogramming your thoughts for success, determining

---

[133] https://www.azquotes.com/quotes/topics/food-medicine.html

why you are on this planet, developing SMART goals and habits, finding faith that frees, moving your body, and incorporating daily support actions such as prayer and meditation.

- Stock a healthy pantry, detoxify your home, support your body with whole-food-based supplements, grow a garden, and mostly, have fun in the process!

If you do all these things, you can go to the doctor and he or she will tell you that you've got a rare condition called good health. You will be an amazing example to your loved ones and to your flock. You will help transform our world by transforming yourself. You truly can be the change you wish to see in the world. Think of the people you love and care about. How can your example encourage them to make the changes they need to restore their bodies, souls, and spirits to a healthy place?

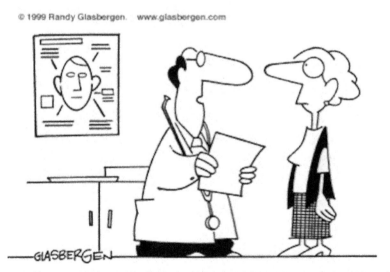

© 1999 Randy Glasbergen.   www.glasbergen.com

"You've got a rare condition called 'good health'.
Frankly, we're not sure how to treat it."

The world is waiting for you to show up in all your amazing authenticity. We need you to make the impact you are meant to make, and to be one hundred percent free (there is no freedom in illness). Make the commitment today to invest in you and your health. Be willing to put your own oxygen mask on first so that you can help others put theirs on. Make you a priority so that you can be around for a long time, God-willing, to leave your mark. You are an amazingly beautiful miracle of God. Don't sit on the sidelines any longer putting off until tomorrow what you can and should do today. I know you've heard it a lot, but today really is the first day of the rest of your life. Make it a great one by knowing how deeply loved you are by your Creator. Love yourself into a healthier you, and joyfully fulfill your purpose! You are worth it!

I hope to someday meet you, but in the meantime, I pray this prayer over you:

"May the Lord bless you and take care of you, may the Lord be kind and gracious to you, may the Lord look on you with favor and give you peace."

Numbers 6:24-26, GNB

ACKNOWLEDGEMENTS

IT'S DIFFICULT TO thank every single person who has ever impacted my life and work, but I would like to express my deepest gratitude to some very special folks, without whom, this book would not be in your hands right now:

- To my husband Tim, my number one cheerleader, best friend, and the love of my life—your belief in me, encouragement, and mostly love, allow me to blossom into who I am meant to be. You bring out the best in me and have taught me more than you can ever imagine. You calm my fears, dry my tears, and make me laugh. I love you beyond words! Thank you for being you and being the wind beneath my wings! And thank you for your contribution in the section on meditation. I have seen the practice transform your life. Thank you for your example!

- To my kids and grandkids—you are the reason I place self-care as a priority. I want to be around as long as possible for you, and to leave you a legacy of health and vitality. I choose to pay whatever price necessary to be the best version of me, so that you will have the courage to be the best version of you. You impact me in ways you don't realize, and each one owns a piece of my heart. I love you!

- To all my siblings—I cannot imagine this life without your love and influence. I extend special kudos to my sisters Karen and Nancy for providing valuable editorial guidance and financial support. We three started this plant-based journey together and have been at it since 1976. I love you!

- To a few of my women armor bearers who were willing to encourage me, pray me through this process, and believe in me when at times I didn't believe in myself— Ramona Pendle, my spiritual mom, mentor, and beautiful friend—your constant encouragement keeps me going when I want to quit. Dr. Carol Watson, my best friend and fellow wellness warrior— our chats each week got me through some very difficult moments in my journey to believe my voice matters. To some of my gal-pals—Ann (my bestie since we were a wee five years-old), Isabel, Glorianne, Sher, Angi, Nancy, Patsy, Lori, Helane, Vasanthi, Celine, and so many more too numerous to mention—your love and friendship mean the world to me!

- Dr. Will Nields—thank you for partnering with me to make a difference in our world. The best is yet to come! Please check out our podcast launching soon titled *Docs UnBoxed* (www.DocsUnBoxed.com) where we will bring you updated and life-changing information to help you flourish!

- To my paternal grandfather, Daddy Doc (Herbert R. Nusz, MD), who practiced medicine the way it was meant to be, using nature whenever possible. Although I barely knew you, your influence and legacy continue as I teach people to use food as medicine and natural-healing principles to heal the body.

- To Rebecca Miles for the cover artwork. You took my vision and painted it beautifully. Your talent knows no bounds. (Check her out at www.vraix.art)

- To the many people who allow me to guide them through my classes, consultations, seminars, and retreats—serving you is an honor!

- And finally, I thank you, the reader—my passion to see you live in peak health is what inspired me to take the time to write this book. I believe in you and your ability to make changes that will help you live longer and better! Take it one step at a time and summit that mountain called Peak Health. You will look back and realize every step was worth the effort, and my guess is you will have had a lot of fun along the way. The best part is you will inspire others as well with your example.

"Example is not the main thing in influencing others. It is the only thing."

Albert Schweitzer

ABOUT DEB HARRELL, ND

DR. DEB HARRELL is a passionate wellness warrior with more than twenty years of experience teaching people how to reclaim their health—body, soul, and spirit. Her inspirational workshops, retreats, and coaching have equipped people to live lives of vitality, passion, and purpose. Deb is a **Naturopathic Doctor** and **Professional Wellness and Lifestyle Coach**. She is a **Certified Health Minister** with Hallelujah Acres Back to the Garden Health Ministry, a **Competent Communicator** with Toastmasters International, and a certified instructor with **Learning Strategies**. She was voted by her peers as **Healthcare Professional of the Year in 2009.** Dr. Deb uses a uniquely holistic approach to wellness including whole-food plant-based nutrition, stress management, lifestyle counseling, and more.

Deb spent fifteen years in accounting management for large and mid-sized corporations while raising her family. As a professional accountant—juggling work, staying healthy, and raising a family—Deb found that she was putting self-care at the bottom of her long to-do list. A duodenal ulcer that resulted was the catalyst to send her on a personal-growth journey that helped Deb discover the solutions that not only brought physical healing, but emotional and spiritual healing as well. Deb offers tried and true simple solutions for busy people! She has spoken internationally on topics of wellness and success to audiences including Nationwide Insurance, the Florida Dental Association's annual conference, numerous organizations, and churches. Deb's passion is to end human and animal suffering caused by food choices! She has been plant-based since 1976. Deb has helped many people heal holistically, including late-stage cancer. Her philosophy is that food is your best medicine. Deb and her husband Tim live in Jacksonville, Florida. They have five grown children and twelve grandchildren. Deb's family is her WHY for making self-care a priority! She wants to create a healthier world for future generations!

CPSIA information can be obtained
at www.ICGtesting.com
Printed in the USA
BVHW091941221221
624600BV00014B/1770